"*Transforming Ethnic and Race-Based Traumatic Stress with Yoga* is filled with beautifully crafted stories that are deeply meaningful and delightful to read. Dr. Parker offers a treasure trove of tools, practices, and life lessons to enhance our yoga practice of Svadhyaya (self-study) to liberate and transform the mind from damaging narratives, both self-imposed and external, and guides us toward the healing power of truth."

—*Jana Long, Executive Director of Black Yoga Teachers Alliance*

"In her latest book, Dr. Gail Parker skillfully weaves a roadmap inspiring radical self-care for reclaiming self-renewal, liberation, and inner peace from the strands of your life, unraveled by the indelible wounds of racial stress and trauma. Compassionately threading timeless Yogic wisdom, affirming-restorative practices, and written reflection equips your inner loom of mindful awareness to continuously unveil the magnificent tapestry of your true authentic nature, a masterpiece of embodied wholeness, clarity, and resilience."

—*Jennifer B. Webb, Ph.D., clinical health psychologist, Associate Professor at UNC Charlotte, yoga and wellness equity researcher, and Advisory Board Member, Give Back Yoga Foundation*

"Gail Parker's previous book was a timely guide to helping us understand and acknowledge race based stress and trauma. *Transforming Ethnic and Race-Based Traumatic Stress with Yoga* is the follow-up we need to actually DO something about it. Race is a delicate conversation, but Parker has the gift of nuance that allows us to understand one another more deeply. If you're willing to unlearn your racial and ethnic stereotypes, prejudices, and biases, read this book and prepare to be transformed."

—*Tamara Jeffries, Senior Editor,* Yoga Journal

"This timely reflection on yoga is a gift for the ages. Dr. Parker personifies the growth, healing, and transformation she advocates and leads the discussion of social change by example. At a time when discussions about race are as violent as action, this book exemplifies working through race in positive and progressive ways."

—*Stephanie Y. Evans, Professor and Director, Institute for Women's, Gender, and Sexuality Studies, Georgia State University, and author of* Black Women's Yoga History: Memoirs of Inner Peace

"TRANSFORMATIVE…HEALING…COLLECTIVE GROWTH. With her first book, Dr. Gail laid the foundation of understanding race-based traumatic stress, but with THIS sequel, she guides the reader on an expedition of therapeutic self-discovery. Whether you are the cause or recipient of race-based traumatic stress, this book with the relatable stories, affirmations, and accompanying yoga asanas is exactly what EVERYONE needs to press forward to radical healing in the form of true transformation. Thank you, Dr. Gail, for your commitment to true and lasting healing."

—*Daheia J. Barr-Anderson, Ph.D., MSPH, Associate Professor of Kinesiology at University of Minnesota, yoga researcher focusing on African-American women, and 250-hour RYT*

Transforming Ethnic and Race-Based Traumatic Stress with Yoga

by the same author

Restorative Yoga for Ethnic and Race-Based Stress and Trauma
Gail Parker
Illustrated by Justine Ross
Forewords by Octavia F. Raheem and Amy Wheeler
ISBN 978 1 78775 185 9
eISBN 978 1 78775 186 6

TRANSFORMING ETHNIC AND RACE-BASED TRAUMATIC STRESS WITH YOGA

GAIL PARKER, PH.D.

ILLUSTRATED BY JUSTINE ROSS

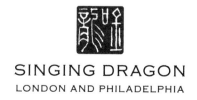

SINGING DRAGON
LONDON AND PHILADELPHIA

First published in Great Britain in 2022 by Singing Dragon,
an imprint of Jessica Kingsley Publishers
An Hachette Company

1

A CIP catalogue record for this title is available from the British Library and the Library of Congress

ISBN 978 1 78775 753 0
eISBN 978 1 78775 754 7

Printed and bound in the United States by West Publishing Corp

Jessica Kingsley Publishers' policy is to use papers that are natural, renewable and recyclable
products and made from wood grown in sustainable forests. The logging and manufacturing
processes are expected to conform to the environmental regulations of the country of origin.

Jessica Kingsley Publishers
Carmelite House
50 Victoria Embankment
London EC4Y 0DZ

www.singingdragon.com

To Growth

CONTENTS

ACKNOWLEDGMENTS

I SHARE my deepest gratitude to those who helped me create this book:

To my editor Sarah Hamlin and the entire Singing Dragon team for their ongoing support of this work.

To all of my teachers, students, patients, friends, colleagues, and dedicated yogis and yoginis who have been an endless source of inspiration and support throughout the process, and who ask the tough questions that keep me on my toes.

To Dr. Paula Kliger, a brilliant psychoanalyst, meditation teacher, colleague, and friend, whose unwavering support I relied on throughout the process of writing this book.

To Nya Patrinos, whose feedback after a workshop I facilitated years ago on Restorative Yoga for race-based traumatic stress opened me to a new dimension of teaching this practice that inspired my approach to writing this book.

To Danielle Graham for her unwavering support of this work and her technical expertise.

To my husband, Dr. Tom Johnson, and my son, Jason Johnson, Esq., my two biggest fans, who continue to inspire and support me and my work. I am grateful for your love and unconditional support.

Thank you all.

Note to the Reader

THROUGHOUT THIS guide I have used the terms "transformation" and "healing," sometimes interchangeably. It was not until reading and re-reading the manuscript that it occurred to me that there is a difference between the two. Healing is a term we use when we discuss illness or injury. Racial stress and trauma are emotional injuries that, left unhealed, become chronic and can lead to negative health outcomes. To that extent, healing the wounds of racial distress is necessary for health and wellbeing. Transformation, on the other hand, suggests change—in this case, positive change that leads to growth. To that end, transformation can be a change agent and can also be the result of healing. Deciding which comes first, or even if that matters, is outside the scope of this book. What is true is that healing the wounds of racial distress along with individual personal and collective transformation are essential to a better quality of life for us all. Yoga is a science, a philosophy, a practice, and an art that can both effect healing and lead to positive transformation.

PROLOGUE

ACCORDING TO Hindu mythology, the Asuras, which simply means not-Suras, and the Suras were neighbors who had various shared and divergent interests. Neither group was particularly interested in interacting with or getting to know the other. Over time, for a complex set of reasons, the Asuras, who were at one time revered as gods, became known as demonic. What started out as different and unknown became confused with "other" in a negative sense. The Asuras came to be described as darker beings, evil spirits, or demons, while the Suras were described as beings of light, as gods. The story of the Suras and the Asuras is ultimately the story of the demonization of "that which is not like me."[1]

Like the Suras and Asuras, we live in a complex world of difference that today, in a positive way, we would call diversity. We are members of a global community, different from each other but not separate. Instead of seeing our own views as the totality of the human experience, yoga offers the view of the human race as one family, each member with his or her own unique contributions, gifts, and talents that need to be tapped, developed, and shared.

We are connected but we are not all the same. We don't look alike, think alike, talk alike, or act alike. But unlike the Suras and Asuras who kept their distance from each other, yoga asks us to join together to get to know, honor, celebrate, and share our perspectives and experiences with each other. It invites us to enter into relationship with that which is unfamiliar and "not like me," even if it makes us uncomfortable. Yoga doesn't ask us to be the same because sameness quickly devolves into conformity. Once that happens, our uniqueness becomes a problem. Even though there is comfort in sameness, a desire for it can be negative because it negates the other person's perspective: "I wish you were like me, not like you."

The negativity of sameness ruptures connection. It prevents us from being all that we can be and from being able to connect authentically with others. There are two forms this negativity can take. The first form is devaluing yourself or someone else. The second form is elevating yourself over someone else. When we regard ourselves as superior to those who are different from us, we deceive ourselves and we annihilate them. When we regard ourselves as inferior to those who are different from us, we in effect annihilate ourselves and deprive others of our genius.

Each one of us is a gift, like a flower that emerges. Our yoga is to engage with our gifts and our experiences and then share them. When drawn together and shared, all of our experiences, gifts, and talents become the opportunity for evolution and growth. In sharing our gifts and our experiences, we discover and strengthen our connection to each other, and we nourish that which is greater than ourselves. We don't have to deny difference to keep from demonizing it. We can accept, honor, and cherish it. Our differences are part of what makes us unique. And while we have different interests and backgrounds, we share a common humanity.

Acknowledging our differences does not have to divide us; in fact, acknowledging our differences can help us develop closer bonds through mutual understanding and respect. Because of differences in national, cultural, gender, racial, ethnic, and religious identity, and due to differences in sexual orientation, ability, age, body size, and learning styles, a person's frame of reference and perspectives may be different from but no less valid than your own. Let us learn and then teach each other to embrace the totality of the human race as one's own people, as members of the human family, no matter who they are or where they come from.

The preconditions of a functional community require that each of us values ourselves and one another. We do this by:

- knowing who we are
- honoring our own uniqueness
- affirming each other's differences
- advocating for each other's reality and potential
- sharing our gifts and talents with each other.

Respect for difference asks that we recognize that different does not mean better than or less than. It is not something to be hated, feared, or eradicated. Different just means different. Rather than demonize difference, yoga invites us to engage, embrace, and celebrate our uniqueness. Yoga means union, the connection of body, heart, and mind, the connection of breath to movement, the connection of one human being to another. It is an invitation to intimacy with oneself and to be in connection with others.

INTRODUCTION

THE TIME FOR POSITIVE CHANGE IS NOW

Ethnic and race-based traumatic stress is real. It is a worldwide phenomenon. Regardless of race and ethnicity, we are all impacted by its damaging effects, from those who are wounded to those who intentionally or unwittingly do the wounding. Othering—the habit of marginalizing or excluding those who do not share your same characteristics—has been historically associated with outbreaks of infectious diseases. During the Covid-19 global pandemic, we are seeing a worldwide uptick in xenophobia and racism. People of Asian descent are being shunned, stigmatized, and scapegoated.[1] And there are reports that just as Asians and people of African descent are being discriminated against in the West, Black African nationals and African Americans have become targets of suspicion, distrust, and racism in parts of China.[2]

In the United States, there are reports that African Americans, Latinx, indigenous communities, and migrants, already at risk due to educational, socioeconomic, and ongoing health disparities, are being denied equal access to shelter, transportation, food, and medical services.[3] The ongoing stress of racial discrimination is a factor that makes African Americans and other non-White communities even more vulnerable to the devastating impact of the global pandemic.[4] Further, there is a large body of evidence that shows that regardless of other factors, including socioeconomic status, race and ethnicity remain significant predictors of a lower quality and intensity of health care and diagnostic services delivered. In the United States, African American, Latinx, and Asian Americans are less likely to receive even routine medical procedures, and one of the contributing factors in the delivery of sub-standard healthcare treatment is the implicit and explicit ethnic and racial bias of healthcare providers.[5] To be clear, beyond other health-related factors, the racial prejudice of healthcare providers is a contributing factor in the health disparities in non-White populations.

Racial and ethnic disparities are not new. But the stress and trauma of physical isolation, or the inability to physically distance from others due to the nature of one's work or living conditions, plus the loss of income, or the loss of life, adds another layer of stress on people who already suffer due to social determinants that discriminate based on skin color, facial features, ethnicity, and racial identity. While pandemics are disruptive and have a negative impact socially, psychologically, and economically, they also create opportunity. Now is an opportunity for progress. We are in the midst of evolutionary change as we witness a global awakening to the pandemic of racial violence and its pernicious effects on all of us. This a pivotal time in our transformation as conscious beings. Events that are unfolding, and our responses to them, have the potential to change each of us for the better. The willingness to change and be changed for the better requires resilience as well as shifts in consciousness. It involves a willingness to recognize that going back to the way things were is not realistic. Accepting reality as it is, with a willingness to envision a brighter future for all, is the opportunity for growth that we are faced with going forward.

Prioritizing mental health is key to tackling the issues associated with race-based traumatic stress for those who perpetuate harm and for those who are harmed. Self-care practices that support psychological health and wellbeing and that promote post-traumatic growth are also necessary. This self-study guidebook is written to support the reduction of the harmful effects of ethnic and race-based traumatic stress so that we can be prepared to create a future that, regardless of one's skin color, facial features, hair texture, and unique cultural, racial, and ethnic identity, embraces the fact that we are all members of the same race—the human race.

As conscious beings, we have a responsibility to recognize racism and xenophobia, to examine our own internalized racial and ethnic biases, and to examine how we have been impacted by racism and xenophobia. Whether or not we know it, like it, or believe it, deeply embedded culturally accepted stereotypes shape our attitudes toward ourselves and others. If we choose to live a conscious life, we can begin by shining a light on our racial and ethnic attitudes and wounds. We can rid ourselves of conscious and unconscious prejudices and shape our consciousness to be open to embrace and celebrate a world that is becoming more varied and expansive every moment. We can examine our biases and challenge their validity. We can identify and recover from unacknowledged and unhealed emotional wounds from the racial violence we have experienced and endured. Being centered and grounded in the core of our being will support us in being able to see clearly and to make choices based on wisdom and compassion, and not on emotions that are influenced by our social conditioning. This is how we change ourselves and create a better future for all.

UNLEARNING RACIAL BIAS

In 2009 the National College Athletic Association (NCAA) premiered a documentary film called *Game of Change* at the iconic March Madness basketball tournament held that year in Detroit, Michigan. The documentary told the story of a historic moment when college basketball ushered in the beginning of the dismantling of racial barriers in college athletics.

> On March 15, 1963, during the middle of the Civil Rights movement, the Ramblers of Loyola University played Mississippi State in a regional semifinal game known as the Game of Change. The unwritten rule in basketball at the time was that only two African American players could be starters. In defiance of the rule, Loyola University's head coach allowed four African Americans to start on the five-man team. In Mississippi, the unwritten law prohibited playing against racially integrated teams. Earlier that season, Loyola had won 20 games back to back which earned them a place in the championship tournament that year. The Game of Change took place at Michigan State University in East Lansing, Michigan. In defiance of an injunction issued by the Governor of Mississippi, that was intended to prevent the game altogether, the all-White Mississippi State team secretly traveled to Michigan to play. Photographers captured one of the great moments in college sports history before tip-off when Loyola captain Jerry Harkness and Mississippi State captain Joe Dan Gold shook hands at center court. As hard as it may be to believe, this was during a time when White people in the United States did not want to be seen having any kind of physical contact with Black people. Loyola won the game by ten points, 61–51, and went on to win the 1963 NCAA Championship.[6]

As part of the March Madness tournament, a select group of ticket holders were invited to an event to view the documentary and then listen to a panel discussion of former professional basketball players, followed by audience discussion. I facilitated the panel and audience discussions. Bill Russell, a former National Basketball Association (NBA) player, was among those on the panel to discuss the film after it was shown. As he discussed the experiences of racism that he and other African American NBA players were exposed to, one of the audience members commented, "We're not racist. We weren't born that way. We learned it." It was a lightbulb moment for me. I remember thinking at the time, if you realize that you have learned to be racist, that the word is not a derogatory term but rather a descriptive one *and* a learned behavior, that means you're capable of realizing that you can unlearn it. If you're willing to unlearn your racial and ethnic stereotypes, prejudices, and biases and be transformed in the process, keep reading.

RACE-BASED TRAUMATIC STRESS IS REAL

There are currently few adequate therapeutic structures in place to help members of communities who face ethnic and race-based stress and trauma throughout their lives to process their experiences. Due to constant exposure, ethnic and race-based traumatic stress is a powerful risk factor for the development of ongoing psychological distress. A Boston College study reports, "Racial trauma is a cumulative experience, where every personal or vicarious encounter with racism contributes to a more insidious, chronic stress."[7] This stress is often magnified by the lack of opportunity to recover before the next experience. To that end, self-study and self-care strategies that lessen the psychological impact and physical toll are needed to manage the ongoing, cumulative, and recurrent stress and trauma of race-related events.

Race-based traumatic stress injury is defined as any external race-related event that causes emotional pain. It refers to experiences of discrimination, threats of harm and injury, humiliating and shaming events, in addition to witnessing harm to other individuals. The incidents are always sudden, unexpected, and uncontrollable, and their occurrence is ongoing, recurrent, and cumulative. The core stressor of ethnic and race-based traumatic stress is emotional pain. The response to the pain is regarded as adaptive, not as pathological. Even though the symptoms are similar, it is distinct from post-traumatic stress disorder (PTSD), which is regarded as a psychiatric disorder caused by a past life-threatening event that leaves the individual unable to shake off the trauma, sometimes even after treatment.

Researchers have made a clear connection between actual and perceived ethnic and racial discrimination and negative health outcomes such as depression, anxiety, insomnia, hypervigilance, headaches, self-blame, self-doubt, shame, body aches, inability to focus, poor memory, and guilt.[8] Preliminary research indicates that mind/body interventions, such as meditation and yoga, are practices that are well suited to be utilized as self-care strategies to empower people to be more involved in their own health care.[9] There is also research that supports the use of positive affirmations as beneficial for stress reduction.[10] And psychologist James Pennebaker discovered in his research that writing about emotionally upsetting events can result in better physical and psychological health.[11] Restorative Yoga and meditation, in combination with affirmations and therapeutic journal writing, offer opportunities to step away from repeated experiences of ethnic and race-based wounding while building the necessary resilience to develop effective coping strategies, and to support post-traumatic growth. For maximum effect, research indicates that Restorative Yoga and meditation should be adapted to be racially, ethnically, and culturally relevant to the populations being served.[12]

SELF-CARE IS HEALTH CARE

Self-care is multidisciplinary and contributes to the overall health of individuals. It involves lifestyle choices that include stress reduction, healthy diet, appropriate rest, adequate exercise, as well as personal growth strategies and spiritual practices. My perspective and approach to self-care as an essential aspect of health is informed by my training and practice as a clinical psychologist and as a lifelong student and practitioner of yoga who integrates yoga, meditation, and psychology as effective therapeutic self-care strategies that enhance emotional balance and physical wellbeing. I base my approach on the biopsychosocial model of health. The model tells us that people experience the world on four different dimensions—the physical, mental/emotional, social, and spiritual levels—and while it may appear that these dimensions are separate, we know that they are not.

The physical dimension is a person's relationship to the material world and the natural environment. It involves embodiment in the world and the relationship to the factual limits and challenges that this presents. The mental/emotional dimension refers to our private relationship to ourselves which is generated by self-reflection and self-study. The social dimension is our everyday relationship to others and includes our relationship to social and cultural norms and lifestyle choices. The spiritual dimension refers to our relationship to the beliefs, ideals, values, and principles that we live by; this dimension determines how we operate on the other dimensions and how we make sense of the world. This perspective was shaped by my undergraduate education in phenomenological existentialism, a philosophical attitude that views human life from one's internal subjective experience rather than pretending to understand it from an outside, "objective" point of view. It is a psychology that emphasizes our creative capacity for self-actualization. My graduate school education in humanistic psychology, an approach that studies the whole person, emphasizing the uniqueness of each individual, and that recognizes each individual's potential for self-actualization, was another powerful influence in shaping my perspective. I have also been influenced by the work of Herbert Benson, MD, a pioneer in the field of mind/body/spirit medicine who supports self-care practices as essential to preventing illness and to maintaining health and wellbeing.[13] Foundational in my approach to this work are the philosophical precepts and practices of yoga as found in Patanjali's Yoga Sutra[14] and the teachings of Paramahansa Yogananda who taught that actualizing the infinite potentials within each of us is yoga's ultimate goal. To that end, yoga is a liberatory practice. The stories I tell and the examples I use are reflective of my lived experience, cultural perspective as an African American woman, and historical context. We each have a story to tell and a perspective that is unique, but the principles shared in this guide are universal and can be generalized to one's own race, ethnicity, cultural conditioning, and historical context.

Yoga regards health as a dynamic continuum that is constantly shifting, varying from day to day, moment to moment. It considers health as the ability to adapt to changing circumstances, to self-manage, and to reach and sustain harmony of the entire human system, body, mind, emotion, and spirit. Health and wellbeing are regarded as qualitative, brought about by living a lifestyle that results in a harmonious homeostatic balance. When body, mind, emotion, and spirit are in harmony, vibrant health is experienced. This involves an understanding of the human system as multidimensional, not just as a physical body.

Yoga offers self-care strategies that help individuals recognize the value of self-awareness and self-regulation as foundational for overall health and wellbeing. The goals of a comprehensive yoga practice include the alleviation of pain and suffering, the prevention of future pain and suffering, and the improvement of overall functioning. Yoga seeks to harmonize all systems of the body, mind, and spirit to attain clarity of mind, inner peace, and freedom from emotional pain and suffering. It is a wholistic approach, that focuses on utilizing codes of conduct (yama and niyama), physical postures (asana), breathing exercises (pranayama), meditation, relevant relaxation techniques, and philosophical precepts as its tools.

According to yoga, dis-ease manifests in the body but originates from states of physical, energetic, mental, emotional, and spiritual imbalance. All five states are interconnected. From a yogic perspective, there is no separation. When all states of being are in balance, wellbeing is experienced. When they are out of balance, symptoms might manifest as emotional disturbance, negative attitudes, physical pain, and disturbed breathing. When the mind is disturbed, it impacts the body; when the body is disturbed, it impacts the mind.

Our state of mind reflects the state of our nervous system, and the state of our nervous system impacts our state of mind. When the nervous system detects threat or picks up cues of danger, it triggers the stress response, more commonly known as the fight–flight response. When the nervous system detects cues of safety, the relaxation response is triggered, causing us to feel calm. Our thoughts come after the nervous system's response, to match whatever feelings of threat or safety we experience, not the other way around. But the nervous system's response, which is outside of conscious awareness, is not always right. It doesn't always know the difference between an external threat or an internal trigger. That's where self-study, clarity of mind, and alert awareness come in. When the nervous system carries unacknowledged stress or unhealed trauma, it can pick up cues of danger where there are none, or cues of safety in dangerous situations. While we do not have control over the nervous system's response, which is automatic and beneath consciousness awareness, we do have control over how we interpret and react to the nervous system's signals. Yoga helps regulate the nervous system, bringing it into a balanced state, making nervous system responses more reliable. Yoga practices help tone the nervous system, aid in preventing and reducing stress, support growth, help restore health and wellbeing, and build resilience. A toned nervous system aids in the ability to identify potential triggers for anxiety, and promotes the ability to discern the difference between an external threat and an internal trigger, bringing conscious awareness to the source of one's problem. When you are consciously aware of the source of any problem you may experience, the likelihood of choosing wise action to solve the problem is increased.

GO WITH THE FLOW

Everything is in a constant state of flux. The body changes, thoughts change, emotions change, motivations change, circumstances and conditions change. Life is a series of natural and spontaneous changes over which we have no control. Struggling against life's inevitable changes creates frustration, sorrow, and stress. Resistance to change is understandable because human beings are attracted to certainty, but a goal of yoga is to soften that resistance and to support individuals in adjusting to and accepting reality as it is. As you learn to let reality be reality, even when it's painful and when things aren't going your way, prana, the life force, flows freely, supporting health and vitality. When we fight reality by holding rigidly to our self-image, our preferences, aversions, and fears, the way things were, or the way we think things should be, we are unable to go with the flow of life, see with clarity, and make wise choices. Yoga teaches us to go with the flow of life as it naturally unfolds, and that inner peace depends on a realistic approach to the uncertainties and fears that are an unavoidable part of life.

WELLBEING IS A CHOICE

Self-care can seem elusive to people who are used to negating their own wellbeing by putting their families, communities, friends, and jobs first. While all emotional pain and suffering cannot be avoided, choosing wellbeing by engaging in self-study and the self-care practices presented in this guidebook can alleviate emotional distress, support resilience, and enhance restoration and growth.

Transforming Ethnic and Race-Based Traumatic Stress with Yoga is a companion to the book *Restorative Yoga for Ethnic and Race-Based Stress and Trauma*. It is intended to have universal appeal across nationalities, cultures, ethnicities, and races. It offers practices that support both psychological and physical health and wellbeing through self-study and self-care practices that anyone can do, and that can weaken the negative effects of ethnic and race-based stress and trauma, whether you are the one being targeted or the one doing the targeting. It aims to remind us that while we may be apart, we are never separate, and that we are only as healthy as our most vulnerable.

We store stress and trauma in our bodies. A popular way of saying this is that the issues are in our tissues. This is why mind/body/spirit approaches to reducing stress and transforming trauma are effective. The guidebook will address all three by presenting practices that can lead to mitigating the emotional wounds associated with ethnic and race-based stress and trauma.

REST IS A SUPERPOWER

When you are steeped in centuries of resisting oppression, active in your community associations, churches, PTAs, and social justice movements, taking care of your children, aging parents, and relatives, forgoing meals, sleep, and personal time to meet all of your responsibilities, you need rest. Rest is not a luxury. It is, in fact, your superpower.

To the extent that you are focused on your activism, resisting racist policies and doing the heavy lifting, you find yourself giving from your depth and not from your overflow, depleting yourself and making yourself vulnerable to burnout and stress-related illnesses. In the face of the Covid-19 global pandemic and the rise in racial violence we are experiencing, we are under more stress than ever. We need our strength as we've never needed it before. We need practices that help us rest and restore our vitality so we can continue our resistance to injustice. We need to center ourselves and our emotional health and wellbeing. We must prioritize self-love and self-care so that we can all live healthier and safer lives. Self-care cannot be an afterthought.

Since we carry our stress and our traumas in our bodies, we need to feel good inside our own skin so that we don't pass on the legacy of racial wounding and our responses to our own unhealed wounds to our children. If you are someone who tends to ignore being stressed, if you are not sure when you are stressed, if you consider yourself a "phenom" because of all that you have accomplished or because of what you do on a daily basis, or if you sometimes wish for a break in your long list of tasks but continue to push anyway, this self-study guidebook can help.

Each of you will have your own experience of what arises as you practice these poses, use the suggested affirmations, and journal. There is no right or wrong experience, and your experience will change each time you engage in the practice. Your cultural, ethnic, and racial identity and your context will influence your experience of these readings and activities. Remember this is an exercise in self-study. For maximum benefit, resist the temptation to attach a desired outcome to the poses, affirmations, and journaling exercises. Expect your experience to change each time you engage in the practice.

Rather than intellectualizing the principles of yoga, this guide will focus on offering you an experience of the teachings. Each chapter will include a reading for your contemplation on an area of ethnic and/or race-related traumatic stress and an illustration of a Restorative Yoga pose, with instructions on how to get into the form of the pose (body), accompanied by a set of relevant affirmations designed to plant seeds of growth in your consciousness. Repeat the affirmations silently while in each pose (mind/emotion). This is followed by a therapeutic journal-writing instruction with blank pages for journal entries to reinforce the affirmations and to identify the psychological, mental, emotional, and spiritual benefits of the posture presented (spirit). Each chapter will follow this format. You can read the chapters sequentially, or choose the chapter that speaks to your immediate need. You can combine postures or just do one at a time. You can choose your own affirmations that may be better suited to you. You can mix and match the affirmations to each posture. This approach is not prescriptive. Listen to your inner guidance and then let the guidebook support you in meeting your need.

Chapter 1

CONSCIOUS LIVING

OUR TASK is not to teach the unconscious to become conscious. Our task is to become aware of and make conscious our own unconscious behavior. Living consciously leads to empowerment.

It means being aware of what goes on around you, what impact you are having on others, and also what goes on in your inner world, of thoughts and feelings. It means noticing and reflecting on what you think about, reflecting on what you feel, being mindful of what you say, and mindful of what you do. Conscious living requires taking the time to pause, breathe, and reflect, making you less reactive, more empathic, more compassionate, and more authentic. Conscious living doesn't just happen. It is intentional and takes effort.

A conscious approach to life is an aware life. It includes being open to more than your own perspective; breaking out of your habitual frame of mind and creating new possibilities; being open to learning and understanding new information instead of protecting and defending what you already know. It leads to welcoming and embracing the unknown. It involves getting to know yourself and others from the inside out.

A conscious life leads to feelings of greater control, freedom of action, and less stress. Being conscious helps us make choices that keep us healthy physically, mentally, emotionally, and spiritually. Being aware of the movements of breath is a portal to conscious living. Life begins and ends with breath. We take our first breath when life begins, and our last breath at the end of life. Breath itself is life and life is breath. We cannot live without it. It is commonly thought that we breathe with our lungs alone. But in truth with each inhale the wave of breath moves through the entire body, beginning deep in the abdomen, inflating the belly, and spiraling upward as the front, side, and back of the body expand. With each exhale, the expiratory wave of breath begins in the upper part of the body and spirals downward as the chest and belly deflate. When we breathe with awareness and intention, we experience the greatest gift of being human—conscious living.

Breath's movements rhythmically ebb and flow like waves in the ocean. Like the sea, the flow of breath may be rapid and turbulent, slow and gentle, shallow or deep. Be still and notice. Your breath is the voice of your body, and the quality of breath is what determines whether or not it is pleasurable. When you focus on your breath, you become attuned to its messages. When it speaks in whispers, like a soft lullaby, soothing and rocking you in its warm embrace, it calms you. When you feel agitated, breath is labored and turbulent, moving rapidly with intensity. Pay attention. Each inhale and exhale tells the story of the natural ebb and flow in all of life. What story is your breath telling you? Breathing easily and fully is one of the basic pleasures of being alive. The breath holds the secret to the highest bliss. It is the dominant factor in the practice of Restorative Yoga. It is a gateway to self-study.

For many, talking about race violates a long-held cultural taboo, and can trigger some defensive responses. But if you take a leap and begin to ask yourself some questions about how you relate to race and ethnicity, the internal barriers that keep you from going deeper into this aspect of self-discovery might soften and begin to dissolve. Awareness of your internalized barriers is the beginning of your personal journey of waking up and living consciously regarding race and ethnicity.

REST

Asana/posture

Studying your breath in a supported Corpse Pose (Savasana) is a good place to begin self-examination. By practicing in stillness and silence, you are able to rest, reflect, and renew without reactivity.

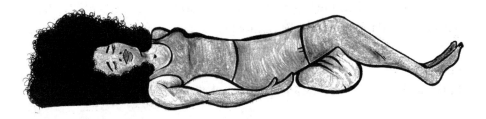

Sit on the floor with your legs slightly bent. Slide a bolster or blanket roll beneath your knees and slowly lower your back, neck, then head onto your yoga mat or blanket. Let your arms rest comfortably by your sides, palms facing up. If you are comfortable doing so, close your eyes or use an eye pillow. Remember in this practice, comfort is key. Become aware of your normal, natural rhythmic breath.

REFLECT

Affirmations

While in the posture, silently repeat to yourself three times, "Breathing in, I feel alive... Breathing out, I feel refreshed." Then on your fourth inhale, silently repeat, "Alive." On your exhale, silently repeat, "Refreshed." Continue that repetition—inhale "Alive," exhale "Refreshed"—for at least five more rounds, and then return your focus to your breath, resting in silence. Notice how you feel.

Rest here for anywhere from five to 20 minutes. When you are ready, roll onto your right side and come into fetal position. Pause here, take two to three breaths, and gently press your hands into the floor to lift back up to seated. Bring your hands toward your heart in prayer position, Anjali Mudra; bow your head slightly toward your heart as you silently offer expressions of gratitude for the benefits of the practice.

Resting in Savasana with a focus on breath teaches that even though breathing is part of our autonomic nervous system, and for the most part goes on automatically and unconsciously, it is the one autonomic function over which we can exercise some control. It teaches us to be aware and conscious of ourselves in ways that we may not always be. It teaches us that we can use our breath to reach a state of equilibrium when we are agitated. It teaches us that we can energize ourselves through breath when we feel lethargic or depleted. It reminds us that we are alive and that we can become renewed when we take the time to be aware of our breath's ability to sustain and support us. Repeating the phrases "I feel alive" and "I feel refreshed" plants seeds that can take root in your consciousness and enable you to regard yourself as vital and energized.

RENEW

Journal

In your journal, finish the sentence "I feel alive and refreshed when..."

_____

_____

_____

_____

_____

_____

_____

_____

_____

_____

_____

_____

_____

_____

_____

_____

_____

_____

_____

_____

Journal how this practice benefits you.

_____

_____

_____

_____

_____

_____

_____

_____

_____

_____

_____

_____

_____

_____

_____

_____

_____

_____

_____

_____

_____

_____

_____

Chapter 2

INNOCENCE

IN THE 1977 television mini-series *Roots*, the true story of the evolution of an enslaved family, there is a scene that left a lasting impression on me. Kizzy, a young girl born and raised in enslavement, is being schooled by her parents about how to speak properly to White people so she doesn't get whipped for saying the wrong thing. While she's listening to her mother and father, she picks up a stick and innocently writes her name on the dirt floor of the family cabin. Both of her parents look frozen in fear. Finally, her horrified mother asks her how she learned to write her name. When Kizzy tells her mother that Missy Ann, the plantation owner's daughter, taught her how to read and write when they used to play school together as younger children, Kizzy's mother slaps her hard across the face and, with a stern look and harsh voice, warns her daughter that by knowing how to read and write, Kizzy risks something worse than being whipped. She risks being sold. She admonishes her daughter, "No reading, no writing ever again." When Kizzy laments that she and Missy Ann won't be able to be friends anymore, Kizzy's mother softens and tells her daughter that she needn't worry about the loss of her childhood friend because "things change" after childhood. She assures her that because she has all the love she needs from her parents, losing Missy Ann as a friend won't matter.

We live in a culture of discipline and punishment that has a double standard for Black and White children, leaving Black children little room for error. But a key characteristic of childhood is immature decision making. Growing up, most of us have experienced being scolded or, worse, punished for our childlike behavior: being too loud, too rambunctious, too curious, messy, or clumsy, talking back, being mischievous—the list goes on. Many of us have been blamed by our parents for things we didn't do and maybe even punished unjustly because they were too tired, stressed, impatient, busy, or distracted to take the time to hear our side of the story. As children, when my brother and I got punished for doing something we didn't do, my mother would always say, "Well, if you didn't do it this time, this is for all the times you did do something wrong that I didn't know about." Case closed. Blessedly, these instances were always softened by the love we knew our parents had for us. It was not until I was much older that I understood that what motivated my parents' harsh and sometimes unfair treatment of us was their fear for our safety. Fear that if my brother and I did not receive harsh punishment at home, that if we were permitted to behave unchecked the way children behave, impulsively, immaturely, and innocently, harm would come to us once we were out in the world, away from their loving protection. Because of our vulnerability to a double standard that they knew existed, which would see us as being guilty of wrongdoing even in our innocence, they came down hard on us.

My cousin, who is now deceased, told a story about a time he was physically punished by his father for being expelled from middle school for fighting. Left alone crying in his room, he overheard his parents arguing about the harshness of the punishment, and he heard his father say to his mother, "Who would you rather do it, me or the police?" This is a style of parenting that mixes fear and love. It is an adaptation that has been passed on from one generation to the next, that believes that harsh punishment is a lifesaving form of love and protection. Physical punishment was an adaptive survival tactic designed to keep children safe during the reign of racial terror of enslavement and Jim Crow. But continuing to use spanking and harsh treatment as necessary forms of discipline outside of that context is maladaptive. Current research shows that harsh punishment has a negative impact on children and does more harm than good.[1]

There is a legacy of racial discrimination and violence in the United States that dehumanizes, "adultifies," and sexualizes Black boys and girls. It influences how they are perceived and how they are treated. By the age of five, Black girls are regarded as being older than they are, as needing less nurturing and protection than White girls, and as being more knowledgeable about sex and other adult topics than White girls.[2] Around the age of ten, Black boys are seen as being four and a half years older than they actually are. Their impulsive, immature, childlike behavior is interpreted as being intentional and malicious.[3] They are seen as being guilty of wrongdoing without ever receiving the benefit of the doubt. Sometimes the results are fatal. Tamir Rice, a 12-year-old boy, was shot and killed by a police officer within seconds of the police officer spotting him playing with a toy gun in a public park. He was described by his assassin as being 20 years old. To justify murdering him, the police officer claimed he feared for his own life. He was never charged with a crime.[4] Contrast this with the treatment of a White male who, at age 17, was driven across state lines by his mother to a community protest that was triggered by the police shooting of Jacob Blake, an unarmed Black man. The teen was seen walking through the crowd, past police, with an assault rifle and was not stopped. It was later determined that he was responsible for shooting and killing two of the protesters and severely injuring another. The following day he was apprehended and placed in juvenile detention, rather than in an adult facility.[5] Compare this with eleven-year-old Nathaniel Abraham, a Black child, who in 1997 became the youngest person on record in the State of Michigan, and perhaps in the United States, to be tried and convicted of murder as an adult. Nathaniel Abraham's attorney is on record saying that he thinks race played a role in the decision, which began a national trend toward putting certain children on trial as adults.[6]

Condemning Black boys and girls for disruptive behavior has implications for how they are treated in schools and by law enforcement. For example, recently, a fifteen-year-old girl, diagnosed with attention deficit hyperactivity disorder (ADHD), was placed on probation for mouthing off and getting into fights with her mother, and for stealing another student's cellphone, which she returned. One condition of the girl's probation was that she complete her school homework assignments. According to her teachers, she was complying and doing well in school, but then with no warning due to the Covid-19 pandemic, her high school abruptly closed and transitioned to remote learning. The teenager was not able to make a quick enough adjustment to online learning, became overwhelmed, fell behind, and stopped completing her homework assignments. Her teacher assured the probation officer that she was helping the student adjust to remote learning and that she did not see the lag in completing homework as a significant problem. The teacher told the probation officer that this student was no farther behind than any of the other students, all of whom were trying to adjust to a new way of learning. The teacher assured the girl's probation officer that she was helping the child make the shift, and that students with different learning styles did better with in-person contact with their teachers, so adjusting to remote learning would take this student a while. Evidently, none of that mattered to the probation officer, or to the judge who ordered the girl to be removed from her mother's home and placed in juvenile detention. Even though she had not committed any offense or broken the law, was getting along well with her mother, and prior to remote learning was doing well in school, she was severely punished.[7] This was a Black girl in an affluent, predominantly White suburban school district and legal jurisdiction. Unlike White children, Black boys and girls aren't as willingly afforded a pass for their youthful lapses in judgment, for their inability to make a quick enough adjustment to change, or for just being children.

A new mother once asked me if I still saw my adult son as my baby. I said, "No. I see him as the man that he is, but I also see his vulnerability and his innocence." I have always seen his innocence, and I always will, but like many parents who know that there is a double standard in the way he will be treated because of the color of his skin, his father and I have been harder on him than he sometimes deserved, as were our parents on us, and their parents before them, and their parents before them. This is how we pass on the legacy of childhood wounding based on our own unrecognized race-based traumatic stress. This is why it is important that we recognize our wounds so as not to pass them on from one generation to the next. Unacknowledged wounds fester and over time can become worse, especially as they lose their original context.

The presumption of guilt begins early in childhood, robbing children of their innocence, causing them to become fearful, overly cautious, and in some cases rebellious. They are forced to grow up too soon. Being given the benefit of the doubt is an example of the presumption of innocence. Blaming the victim, the one who is actually hurt by racial insensitivity, ignorance, or violence, is how victimizers project their shame onto those they harm. An example of projecting shame onto others is the belief that if someone is harmed in any way, they must have done something to cause it or deserve it. That way of thinking blames others for doing something wrong when they have not, and, worse, often teaches us to blame ourselves for the wrongdoing that others inflict on us. One of the most stunning examples of this was a recent experience I had in a social justice and yoga workshop where in a discussion on the concept of karma, the understanding that each and every action has a consequence, the statement was made that individuals who have known systemic oppression were born into this life to experience such things because of their actions in previous lives. This misinformed interpretation of karma is based on the karma theory of the Indian caste system that justified relegating dark-skinned Indians to the lowest caste, and blaming their past-life transgressions on the caste they were relegated to.[8] "This hierarchical ordering of the society, based on karma theory and caste system, was unjust and heartless, bringing untold sufferings to the lower castes and out castes, for thousands of years."[9] After taking several deep breaths and deciding how I wanted to respond, I offered another perspective. I suggested that the presenter and the participants consider that instead of being a punishment, those who have the greatest challenges have them because they have a higher calling, and not because they deserve to be punished. When you are deprived of the presumption of innocence, you internalize feelings of guilt or wrongdoing. This unearned guilt carries over into adulthood and, without conscious awareness, is passed on. A standard of perfection that can never be achieved results, leading to ongoing stress and self-doubt. We need to be conscious of our racial wounding and conscious of the wounding we inflict on others in order to transform its damaging effects.

Dark-skinned children are not the only ones who lose their innocence based on racial prejudice. Have you ever wondered what impact racially prejudiced remarks have on White children? A participant in a seminar I attended told of her experience of "losing her innocence" when she discovered that her mother held racist views and stereotyped people of different races and ethnicities. When she was ten years old her best friend, who was of South Asian descent, invited her to come to her home to play. When she told her mother about the good time she had at her friend's house, her mother asked her in a mocking tone of voice, "Did their house smell like curry?" She said she didn't know what curry was, but it was clear to her that her mother's question was disparaging and a putdown of her friend. She realized her mother thought there was something disdainful about her friend's culture that was worthy of mockery. Even though she didn't fully understand it, she said she felt ashamed of her mother's feelings. She doesn't share her mother's views but said she still carries some of the shame she felt as a child.

Earned guilt is not the same as unearned guilt. Earned guilt is the feeling of shame that comes from causing harm to others. It is actually an emotion that comes from violating your own ethics or moral standards. If you don't regard being abusive toward others as a personal ethical violation, you won't feel guilt, which is why abusers don't feel guilt or shame. When you don't feel shame or guilt, it's easy to be abusive. As unpleasant a feeling as it is, the ability to feel shame puts the brakes on abusive behavior. In this respect shame is actually a good thing. In yoga, the five ethical principles that guide behavior toward others are non-harming or ahimsa, truthfulness or satya, non-stealing or asteya, moderation or brahmacharaya, and non-attachment or aparigraha. When we violate these principles, our guilt tells us that we have done something that goes against our values and signals us to take a different course of action, or to make amends for our transgressions. Being able to tell the difference between earned and unearned guilt can be tricky, especially when you have been acculturated to take responsibility for harm that you may not have inflicted, or to blame those who have been harmed for having done something wrong. This is where our practices come in. It takes intention to become consciously aware of the source of the guilt or shame you feel. It takes time and effort to overcome any unearned guilt you may be carrying. It takes commitment and courage to overcome and make amends for any guilt you have earned by violating the ethical standards that you value.

REST

Asana/posture

Practicing child's pose (Balasana) can serve as a reminder of one's childlike innocence and supports the embodiment of a sense of safety in one's vulnerability, a much-deserved experience for people who have been deprived of resting in safety as children, and a necessary experience for those who are confronting, maybe for the first time, transgressions they have previously ignored. For those who have wittingly or unwittingly caused harm to others, this pose might bring up unpleasant memories of ways you may have violated the five ethical principles of behavior toward others, but this discomfort is a necessary part of the process of change. Love yourself. Reclaim your innocence.

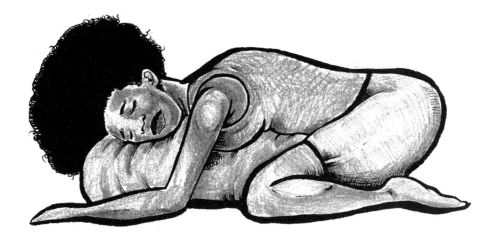

Create a support of firm pillows, blankets, or a bolster lengthwise in front of you. Lower yourself onto your hands and knees, placing them on either side of the support, knees open wide toward the edges of your mat, tops of feet flat on the floor behind you with big toes touching. Sit back on your heels and without lifting your hips, fold your torso forward over the length of the bolster or blankets. Place your forearms and the palms of your hands flat on either side of the bolster, or, if it is more comfortable, bend your elbows and interlace your fingers around the top edge of the support. Turn your head to one side or the other, resting on your cheek, or rest your forehead on the bolster—whichever is most comfortable. Let gravity pull your legs and hips toward the earth as you soften your lower back and release your tailbone toward your heels. Halfway through, turn your head to the other side as your body continues to settle into the pose.

REFLECT

Affirmations

While in the posture, silently repeat to yourself three times, "Breathing in I feel innocent... Breathing out I feel free." On your fourth inhale, silently repeat, "Innocent." On your exhale, silently repeat, "Free." Continue that repetition—inhale "Innocent," exhale "Free"—for at least five more rounds, and then return your focus to your breath, resting in silence. If your head is turned to the side, gently turn it to the opposite side, continuing to focus on your breath and resting in stillness. Hold this pose for five to ten minutes on each side. When you are ready to come out of this pose, take two or three deep breaths and gently press both hands into the floor to lift up to sitting on your heels.

Practicing child's pose can evoke experiences of innocence and has the potential to replace feelings of unearned guilt as the experience of innocence becomes embodied. Repeating the phrases "I feel innocent" and "I feel free" plants seeds that can take root in the consciousness of an individual, enables one to realize the difference between earned and unearned guilt, and supports a compassionate approach to making mistakes and errors in judgment that one is bound to make. Embodying innocence is a form of ahimsa.

RENEW

Journal

In your journal, finish the sentence "I feel innocent and free when..."

_____

_____

_____

_____

_____

_____

_____

_____

_____

_____

_____

_____

_____

_____

_____

_____

_____

_____

_____

Journal how this practice benefits you.

_____

_____

_____

_____

_____

_____

_____

_____

_____

_____

_____

_____

_____

_____

_____

_____

_____

_____

_____

_____

Chapter 3

FORGIVENESS

YOU CAN'T un-spill the milk is a lesson my parents drummed into us as children. They taught us to be mindful of what we thought about, what we said, what we wrote, or what we did because they knew that once a thing is said or done, it cannot be unsaid or undone. We've all said and done things we regret and wish we could take back. How many times have you thought about what you would say or do differently if you could just get a do-over? The thing is, even though life gives us plenty of opportunities to begin again—we call them second chances—it doesn't give us do-overs. Once a thing is done, it's done. I remember being in a grocery store and watching a mother discipline her young child for some transgression. He was crying and from the depth of his little being proclaiming, "Mommy, Mommy, I'm sorry, I'm sorry, I'm sorry." His mother, unmoved by the apology, said with great conviction, "Don't tell me! Show me!" This is where being mindful and living consciously comes in. Has someone ever done something that really hurt you and then did everything within their power to make amends, to show you they regretted their behavior? Were you able to forgive them? When someone does apologize, how do you forgive them? And should you?

I tell a story in the book *Restorative Yoga for Ethnic and Race-Based Stress and Trauma* of an experience I had in a yoga class where the instructor's playlist included a song with the "n" word in the lyrics. After the experience, I didn't think I would ever be able to return to the place that I had trusted and regarded as my yoga home. I didn't want to go back and didn't intend to. But on top of being hurt and angry, I was really sad. The studio owner did everything in her power to make amends. There was nothing more she could do or say that would have communicated her sincerity in making sure that I felt like a valued member of the community. In spite of her sincere apologies, it wasn't enough to make me want to return to the studio. I needed some time. When my husband, seeing how sad I was and how much I missed practicing in the studio, suggested that I consider forgiving what had occurred and return, I resisted. "Why should I do that?" I yelled back. "Because you really love it there and you miss it," he reminded me. He was right. As I sat with my resistance, I was shocked to discover that I didn't want to forgive. I wanted to hold a grudge. I wanted to be mad. Have you ever felt that way?

Anger is a defense against feeling the hurt of being devalued. It can be functional when it's mobilized in a positive direction. To that extent, it serves a useful purpose. It can motivate you to confront a racially charged situation head on, which I had done at the time the hurtful event occurred. But carrying the anger as a grudge weighs you down and keeps you stuck in the past. Dwelling on past grievances is a form of emotional and mental clutter and keeps you from getting on with your life. I knew that my unwillingness to let go of the hurt I felt would do me more harm than good. My grandmother used to say that holding a grudge was like drinking poison and hoping the other person would die. Ultimately, I chose forgiveness, but it was so hard to do. This begs the question, "What baggage are you carrying from past emotional wounds that you should have released a long time ago?"

Forgiveness is not excusing, condoning, justifying, accepting, forgetting, or just moving on from hurtful race-related events, but it is an important step toward letting go of past offenses. It releases you and the other person. It creates opportunities for new possibilities either to form new relationships or to transform old ones. Refusing to forgive keeps you stuck in a cycle of hurt and anger even if you end the relationship. You need to forgive the person who betrayed you before you can let the relationship go, but you don't have to do it in person; instead, you have to do it in your heart. Once you've forgiven someone in your heart, if you still want to forgive them in person, go right ahead. If you need to reconnect with someone so you can begin again, forgive the person first and then push the reset button. When it comes to asking for forgiveness, I'm not a fan because it requires the person you've hurt to focus on helping you feel better about what you did to hurt them, and that's not okay. It robs them of their ability to determine whether or not they want to forgive you, and if so, when. Forgiveness takes time. If you regret having hurt someone, admit what you've done wrong, first to yourself and then, instead of defending what you said or did that was harmful, validate the experience of the person you've hurt, then change your behavior.

FORGIVE YOURSELF

Forgiveness doesn't happen all at once. It is a process that requires regular and consistent practice. If you are having difficulty forgiving someone who you feel has wronged you, start the process by forgiving yourself. Admit it—most of the time when someone has done us wrong, we not only blame them for the wrongdoing, but we blame ourselves for not being smart enough to have avoided the offense. "How could I have been so blind?" "Why didn't I see that coming?" "What I should have done or said instead was…" "Why am I letting this bother me so much?" "Why do I care?" Instead of blaming, shaming, or criticizing yourself for feeling a certain way, for something you wish you hadn't said or done, or for something you wish you had done differently, instead of denying your hurt or pushing it out of conscious awareness, try forgiving yourself using this four-step process:

1. Identify what it is you feel you've done wrong or neglected to do right.
2. Allow yourself to feel the remorse that comes from having done something you regard as wrong or wish you had done differently.
3. Set an intention that you won't repeat the behavior.
4. If you do it again, repeat the first three steps of the forgiveness process and then don't do it again.

We start with self-forgiveness because one effect of ethnic and race-based traumatic stress is the tendency to blame oneself for feeling wounded or hurt or for not avoiding or stopping the painful race-related event. We all have regrets about what we should have felt or what we could have done differently, but it is important that we go easy on ourselves and forgive ourselves. As you practice forgiving yourself, you discover that forgiving others becomes easier. Forgiveness is an important practice when it comes to recovering from race-based stress and trauma.

WHEN NO ONE APOLOGIZES

But what about the hurts that no one apologizes for? In the absence of an apology, how do you move on? Without an apology, how do you forgive? Forgiveness is more for your benefit than for anyone else's. You don't have to receive an apology from someone in order to forgive them, although that sometimes makes it easier. Attaching your ability to forgive to someone else's willingness to apologize gives them your power. Forgiveness itself is a powerful choice. It is an action, a practice, and a process, not an outcome. It doesn't mean putting the past behind you and moving on. It means that you commit to working on healing your wounds by taking good care of yourself, just as you would if you were physically hurt. When you regard forgiveness as a choice to let go of pain and suffering, and an action, not a feeling, the power is in your hands to recover from any damage that was done. You don't have to wait for an apology to forgive.

Forgiveness applies to the big hurts and unspeakable atrocities of racial violence and injustice as well as to the daily recurrent micro-aggressions that people endure. Here's the question. Will you choose it? And then, will you do it? The willingness to forgive can create something very powerful. It can renew depth, intimacy, and new possibility in all of your relationships. It can also free you from relationships that you have outgrown or that you no longer wish to continue.

1. Make a list of people you would like to forgive. How did they hurt you?
2. Make a list of people you have hurt whose forgiveness you long for. How did you hurt them?
3. Allow yourself to feel the regret, remorse, and sorrow that follow.
4. Going forward, make a sincere promise to avoid being hurtful or to avoid holding on to past hurts.
5. Once you've done your forgiveness work internally, if it seems like a good idea to approach the person directly to either forgive them or to make amends for your actions, do it.

The act of forgiveness is like stepping onto your yoga mat. Some days you just don't feel like it but you do it anyway and end up feeling better. The same is true with forgiveness. Some days you just don't feel like it. But do it anyway. Holding a grudge is way overrated. Leave the past where it belongs, in the past.

As Jack Kornfield reminds us, "Forgiveness is giving up all hope for a better past."[1] Contemplate that. Practice forgiveness. Step into the present moment. Instead of wishing for a do-over, let bygones be bygones and then begin again.

REST

Asana/posture

Practicing a supported pigeon pose (Salamba Kapotasana) requires a level of awareness that other postures may not. You cannot throw yourself into this posture. In order to keep from hurting yourself, you must be methodical and mindful of your alignment. This pose can support you in recognizing how gentle you need to be with yourself. The same is true of how you relate to others. If you don't approach others mindfully with sensitivity, you can injure them even if you don't mean to. Remember there is intent and there is impact. We don't intend to hurt ourselves in our yoga practice, but if we are not mindful, we can. We may not intend to be hurtful of others, but if we're not mindful, we can be. This posture also helps you learn the difference between discomfort and pain. Growth can be uncomfortable, especially when you discover things about yourself that conflict with your assessment of who you are, or who you think you should be. But the discomfort of discovery is healing and is not the same as the pain of injury. This posture helps you embody that awareness.

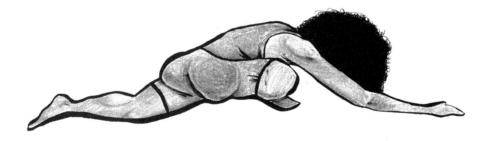

This illustration is the full expression of the posture. To make it restorative, place a bolster or stack of blankets vertically in front of you to support your torso and head, or horizontally in front of you to support your head when you fold forward. Place a block, cushion, or pillow underneath the hip of the front leg to level your hips.

Starting on hands and knees, place the bolster or blanket stack vertically out in front of you. Draw your right knee to your right wrist and pivot your right foot over to the left as you lengthen your left leg back behind you. To protect your bent knee, the heel of your right foot should be close to your left groin. For maximum comfort, place a folded hand towel or other soft folded cloth on the shin of the leg that is extended back behind you.

Before you lower your body or your head onto the bolster in front of you, make sure your hips are level and rest the top of your foot that is extended back behind you flat on the mat. With your hands still on the ground to support you, inhale and lift up out of your waist and fold forward over the bolster as you exhale. Once you feel supported by the bolster, rest your forearms and hands on the mat alongside the bolster and soften your shoulders. Turn your head in the same direction as your extended leg. Take your time getting into this pose. You should feel no sensation in your knee and only mild sensation in your right hip.

Let the bolster hold the weight of your upper body. To transition to the other side: slowly come to hands and knees and stretch one leg back at a time. When you are ready, come back into hands and knees pose and follow the same instruction for the left side. Hold this pose, breathing slowly, for four to seven minutes on each side.

REFLECT

Affirmations

While in the posture, silently repeat to yourself three times, "Breathing in I feel forgiven... Breathing out I feel forgiving." On your fourth inhale, silently repeat, "Forgiven." On your exhale, silently repeat, "Forgiving." Continue that repetition—inhale "Forgiven," exhale "Forgiving"—for at least five more rounds, and then return your focus to your breath, resting in silence. Repeat the affirmations on each side.

A supported pigeon pose is a pose that teaches you to be patient and gentle with yourself. Many of us hold a great deal of tension in our hips and shoulders. Getting into and out of this posture requires that we are mindful and that we treat ourselves with tender loving care. You cannot do this posture quickly and you may not be able to hold it for long, but it teaches you that if you stay with the process, even when it's difficult at first, you will begin to experience the joy of release and of letting go. Then all you have to do is receive the benefits. The process of forgiveness is the process of letting go. Repeating the phrases "I feel forgiving" and "I feel forgiven" plants seeds that support the process of letting go of grievances, guilt, and shame.

RENEW

Journal

In your journal, finish the sentence "I feel forgiven and forgiving when..."

_____

_____

_____

_____

_____

_____

_____

_____

_____

_____

_____

_____

_____

_____

_____

_____

_____

_____

_____

_____

Journal how this practice benefits you.

_____

_____

_____

_____

_____

_____

_____

_____

_____

_____

_____

_____

_____

_____

_____

_____

_____

_____

_____

_____

_____

_____

_____

Chapter 4

BOTTOMS UP

IN A culture that requires working twice as hard to get half as far, and that emphasizes being the best, having the best, and doing the best, ordinary is not what most of us want to be identified with. In an age of celebrity, we dream of being superheroes and superstars. The emphasis on being extraordinary is indicative of a serious imbalance. It's not the desire to be exceptional that is troublesome, it is the belief that you have to be outstanding or exceptional all the time and that if you're not, then you're inferior, not good enough, or, even worse, nobody.

The fact is, our ordinariness is what grounds us and roots us in our humanity. It connects us to one another and gives us a sense of belonging. Contrary to popular belief, it does not deprive you of your individuality. Yoga teaches us that we are both ordinary and unique simultaneously. When we ignore one or the other, we are at risk of being one-dimensional and off balance. Finding the midline between ordinary and extraordinary eases the burden and anxiety of being only one or the other. In the movie *Black Panther*, we see the superheroes display both their ordinary vulnerability and their extraordinary superheroic strength in combination, to demonstrate the depth and complexity of being human.

Poet Lucille Clifton writes about discovering her ordinariness in her poem "the thirty eighth year":

the thirty eighth year
of my life,
plain as bread
round as a cake
an ordinary woman.

an ordinary woman.

i had expected to be
smaller than this,
more beautiful,
wiser in afrikan ways,
more confident,
i had expected
more than this.

i will be forty soon.
my mother once was forty.

my mother died at forty four,
a woman of sad countenance
leaving behind a girl
awkward as a stork.
my mother was thick,
her hair was a jungle and
she was very wise
and beautiful
and sad.

i have dreamed dreams
for you mama
more than once.
i have wrapped me
in your skin
and made you live again
more than once.
I have taken the bones you hardened
and built daughters
and they blossom and promise fruit
like afrikan trees.
i am a woman now.
an ordinary woman.

in the thirty eighth
year of my life,
surrounded by life,
a perfect picture of
blackness blessed,
i had not expected this
loneliness.

if it is western,
if it is the final
europe in my mind,
if in the middle of my life
i am turning the final turn
into the shining dark
let me come to it whole
and holy
not afraid
not lonely
out of my mother's life
into my own.
into my own.

i had expected more than this.
i had not expected to be
an ordinary woman[1]

I suppose most of us, at least some of the time, expect to be more than ordinary, but this poem invites us to actually reflect on our ordinariness. We don't have to give up excellence as a value, but going deeper into the contemplation of ordinary reveals that it has much to offer.

Paying attention to the ordinary means paying attention to the everyday-ness of life—the failures, challenges, and hardships you face, as well as those things that give you pleasure like a delicious home-cooked meal, your favorite Miles Davis album, connecting with friends and family, offering a kind word to someone, walking down a garden path, noticing a cloud formation, a sunrise, or the change of seasons. Observing the mundane aspects of life helps us avoid the shallowness of living a one-dimensional, self-centered life of privilege or of pain. Our very soul is rooted and grounded in the enjoyment of ordinary pleasures.

There's a funny thing about ordinary. When you embrace it in its apparent simplicity, you discover its intricacy, depth, and complexity. We tend to ignore the ordinary because we're used to it. Because it doesn't stand out, we don't put the extra effort into acknowledging it. When we ignore the ordinary, we overlook the value of simple pleasures. Without the ordinary, the extraordinary is meaningless. You really can't have a full life without both. They are not opposites. They are yoked.

Live from your heart and embrace life's deep and ordinary pleasures. When you do these simple acts, true beauty in everything rises to the surface and the ordinary becomes the extraordinary. Embracing the ordinary is not exotic, awesome, or amazing, but it is a recipe for good living and a practical, down-to-earth philosophy of life. When we embrace the ordinary, we become more accepting of others' foibles and of our own. Embracing the ordinary invites us to deal with our daily lives, our successes, our failures, and our mediocrity without having to be perfect. It teaches us to relax, enjoy life, and have fun. Let's turn our perspective upside down and embrace the ordinary as having as much value as the extraordinary. John Lewis advised us that "Ordinary people with extraordinary vision can redeem the soul of America by getting in what I call good trouble, necessary trouble."[2] Learn to value and embrace the ordinary.

REST

Asana/posture

Practicing an inverted posture like legs up the wall (Viparita Karani) supports reorienting and re-envisioning, a new way of being. Being upside down in a posture can help restore equilibrium, while allowing you to remain grounded as you explore a different perspective. Bottoms up.

To perform this receptive inversion, start by sitting on the floor against a wall, knees slightly bent, feet flat on the floor with your right shoulder, hip, and thigh against the wall. Place your hands flat on the floor hip distance apart and slightly behind your hips, fingers facing forward. Begin to lower yourself onto your back, bending your elbows back behind as you swing your legs up the wall. Once your legs are up the wall, scoot your hips as close to the wall as is comfortable. Keep a bolster, or a folded blanket in a rectangular shape, within reach. Bend your knees, press the soles of your feet into the wall, lift your hips, and slide the bolster or blanket underneath them. Straighten your legs and extend them back up the wall. Extend your arms out to the sides, palms facing up, if comfortable, or place your arms in cactus position. If you choose cactus position, lift your arms out to the sides of your body in the shape of a "T" at shoulder height. Bend your elbows to 90 degrees. Keep your upper arms horizontal and bend your forearms back behind you until the backs of your hands are flat on the ground.

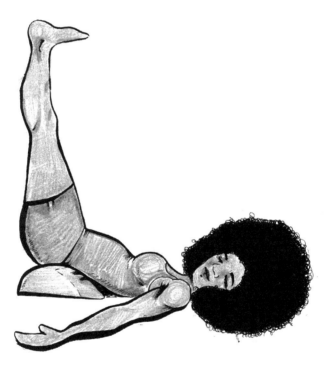

If extra support is needed, place a small neck roll (made from a hand towel, for example) under your neck to support and lengthen the cervical spine.

REFLECT

Affirmations

While in the posture, silently repeat to yourself three times, "Breathing in, I feel rooted... Breathing out, I feel grounded." On your fourth inhale, silently repeat, "Rooted." On your exhale, silently repeat, "Grounded." Continue that repetition—inhale "Rooted," exhale "Grounded"—for at least five more rounds, and then return your focus to your breath, resting in silence. Rest in this pose for up to 15 minutes. When you're ready, bend your knees and press the soles of your feet into the wall, and lift your hips to slide the bolster out from under you. Gently lower your pelvis to the floor, and with your knees still bent, roll to the right side, walking your feet down the wall, and come into fetal position. Pause here, enjoy your breath, tuck in your chin, and use your hand to press yourself back up to sitting.

This supported inverted posture gives you an experience of being able to orient yourself when you are upside down. Race-based traumatic stress is sudden, unexpected, and uncontrollable. It always throws you for a loop. Learning to rest in this upside-down pose is good practice for learning how to regroup and reorient when you are thrown a curve ball. Repeating the phrases "I feel rooted" and "I feel grounded" plants seeds that can take root in your consciousness and enable you to regain your composure even when there is an unexpected event.

RENEW

Journal

In your journal, finish the sentence "I feel rooted and grounded when..."

_____

_____

_____

_____

_____

_____

_____

_____

_____

_____

_____

_____

_____

_____

_____

_____

_____

_____

_____

_____

_____

Journal how this practice benefits you.

_____

_____

_____

_____

_____

_____

_____

_____

_____

_____

_____

_____

_____

_____

_____

_____

_____

_____

_____

_____

_____

_____

_____

Chapter 5

FREEDOM

M Y FATHER'S mother was a proud, dignified, private woman of few words. She expressed herself through her art. Her home on the South Side of Chicago, where she and my grandfather raised six children, was decorated with Victorian-style furniture; her china cabinet was filled with beautiful vintage tea cups and saucers, and scattered throughout the house were artistic boxes of all shapes and sizes filled with all manner of fun things to examine: antique buttons, fancy hair combs, crystals, stick pins, hat pins, and various other trinkets and whatnots. The thing I remember most, though, was the spinning wheel and the loom that sat in her parlor. The spinning wheel was a device that she used to magically turn fiber into thread for sewing or into yarn for knitting or crocheting sweaters, caps, scarves, or blankets. Next to the spinning wheel was a loom that she used for weaving the spun yarn into cloth that she would then use to create afghans, table linens, throws, and decorative wall hangings. Watching her spin and weave was hypnotic.

My grandmother's complexion was very light and she had long, straight, snow-white hair that she braided and fastened on top of her head with fancy hair combs. At night she would let me brush her hair when she took the braids out. When I asked her why her hair was so straight and long, unlike my short, bushy, texturized hair, she said, "I don't know, because there's been no 'White blood' in our family for years." That answer confused me because I didn't know what "White blood" was, or what it had to do with my question, and I was afraid to ask. When I told my mother what my grandmother said, she explained that during enslavement, White slave owners raped their Black female slaves, impregnated them, and then held their own children in bondage. To admit to having "White blood" was to admit to having been born of rape, which to my grandmother and women of her generation was a shameful admission. She learned secrecy and denial as a way to protect herself from feeling that shame.

How many of you grew up in a household where secrecy was the rule, not the exception? "What goes on in this house, stays in this house." It is not uncommon in families with a history of racial trauma for secrecy to be the norm. Secrets are those things we don't want others to find out about, so we keep them hidden. Sometimes secrecy is necessary. Remember the story of Kizzy who had to keep her knowledge of reading and writing a secret to avoid being beaten or sold away from her family? During the era of enslavement, secrecy was also necessary to protect the lives of people seeking freedom from bondage, and to protect the lives of those who helped them escape. In order for any kind of resistance efforts to be successful, secrecy was an absolute necessity. Learning to hide one's feelings was also a necessary strategy to keep people who meant to do you harm from knowing what you really thought, or to keep them from taking advantage of your vulnerabilities. Under life-threatening circumstances, secrecy has value.

Secrecy becomes problematic when it is used habitually and automatically, without context or awareness, and regardless of the circumstances. My grandmother's secrecy was a defense against reigniting the emotional pain of what she regarded as a shameful admission. She learned it from her mother and her grandmother. To this day, there are family stories I will never know on both my mother's and father's sides because of how guarded they all learned to be and because of the secrets they kept. They taught us how to keep secrets, too. We learned not to ask too many questions about their past, and we learned to keep our painful stories to ourselves. We did not tell them about the racial wounding we endured. We suffered in silence, hiding our wounds as they did, never telling our stories. I feel that as a deep sense of loss right now. There is so much I wish I knew but never will because of the silence.

The problem with keeping secrets is your wounds remain hidden. You learn to just keep pushing your feelings and your memories out of your conscious awareness. But here's the thing. Just because the pain of the trauma you have experienced is out of your conscious awareness does not mean it isn't there. It is. It's just hidden beneath the surface and, from time to time, it seeks release and explodes out into the open, like a pressure cooker releasing steam. It usually happens unexpectedly and can leave you feeling regret about any collateral damage your outburst may have caused. Carrying around secrets costs you peace of mind, happiness, and even your health. Keeping secrets interferes with your ability to be yourself, and to be intimate with others. Hiding parts of your personal history takes energy and is stressful. Ongoing stress poses a health problem due to increased hormone levels that cause inflammation and compromise the immune system. These are some of the reasons that keeping secrets is a toxic practice. On top of negative health consequences, when you are unable to process and recover from stressful and traumatic race-related events because you're hiding them, you risk passing on the legacy of your unaddressed, unacknowledged wounds to your children.

Most of us have thoughts, feelings, ideas, dreams, and stories that we've never told anyone. Whether it's an embarrassing story or a family skeleton, each of us has a hidden place within that only we know about. This is our private self. The private self is the part of you that creates boundaries around what you choose to share with others and who you choose to share the most vulnerable parts of yourself with. The private self is the self that fantasizes, daydreams, and holds sacred your deepest beliefs, values, and those things you only share with the ones you trust the most. The private self is conscious, accessible, and intentional. The secret place I'm talking about is different from your private self. Secrets are those things hidden from awareness because of a fear of what may happen if you share them, a fear about what people may think of you, or the shame or fear you might feel if they are exposed. We can begin to break the chains of bondage that secrecy imposes, and address the challenge of truly valuing ourselves by sharing our stories with one another, the ones we've been ashamed to tell, like my grandmother who was ashamed of admitting to having White ancestors. We are held captive by the stories that we keep secret. But blessedly times are changing. Now people are speaking up and speaking out about what was previously unspeakable.

In a 2020 opinion article in *The New York Times* titled "You Want a Confederate Monument? My Body Is a Confederate Monument," poet Caroline Randall Williams writes:

> I have rape-colored skin. My light-brown-blackness is a living testament to the rules, the practices, the causes of the Old South… My skin is a monument… I am a black, Southern woman, and of my immediate white male ancestors, all of them were rapists. My very existence is a relic of slavery and Jim Crow.[1]

She wrote the article in response to the vocal objections and active protests to removing monuments to the legacy of the Southern states that fought in a war to preserve the system of slavery in the United States. This is a woman who is not hiding her story. She is not ashamed of her ancestry. She is speaking her truth and telling her story in all of its rawness. Her healing becomes all of our healing. Even if it's uncomfortable, telling the truth and sharing our stories is where healing begins, not only as individuals, but also as a collective.

But there is more to us than our fear, anger, and shame. We have stories to tell of love, excellence, triumph, courage, and heroism. It's time for us to share all of ourselves with each other—our vulnerability as well as those parts of us that are secure and confident. It is time to free ourselves from the prison of emotional pain and suffering that keeping silent imposes on us, making us feel isolated and alone or like imposters.

It doesn't matter what your story is. Keeping it a secret can cause harm to you physically, psychologically, and spiritually, and can cause harm to others, too. Yoga teaches us that truthfulness, satya, is a guiding principle of our practice both on and off our yoga mat. We learn that by shining a light on the hidden places within ourselves we can safely avoid their stress-related and harmful consequences. Even though the thought of revealing your stories can seem scary, once you take that first step, it becomes easier.

When you're preparing to be open with others about a story you've never shared, a good first step is to stop hiding the truth from yourself. Journal, write a poem, draw a picture, or even write a song about it. If you've been hiding the truth from someone else and you want to open up to them, before you share it with that person, try role-playing what you'll say with a trusted friend first. If you don't feel comfortable divulging the story to someone you know, seek help from a professional who is obligated to maintain confidentiality. There is no shame in seeking counseling.

Being able to share more of yourself helps you become more comfortable in your own skin. By trying to keep your personal history a secret, you are actually repressing other parts of yourself. Years of holding yourself back will cause you to lose touch with who you really are, and will undermine any chance for lasting joy and deep happiness. By sharing your stories in a safe place with a safe person, you will learn to be more open with your family and friends. You'll talk more freely about your past when it comes up.

Don't be imprisoned by your secrets or by the fear of breaking the "What goes on in this house, stays in this house" rule. Don't be imprisoned by your past. There's a story about a baby elephant living in captivity, who was tied to a tree with a rope to keep her from getting away. Because it is the nature of elephants to roam free, the baby elephant instinctively tried, with all her might, to break free from the rope and pull away from the tree. She just wasn't strong enough. After failing time and time again, she gave up the struggle and stopped trying altogether. Once the elephant was fully grown, even though she could have easily freed herself by uprooting the tree and breaking the rope, she no longer made any effort. Since her mind had been conditioned from infancy that she was not free to roam, she had internalized and accepted the boundaries and limitations created by her past. Don't let your past or your secrets keep you in bondage. Here are some suggestions that can help make sharing your secrets a positive experience:

- Be discerning. Choose people who are trustworthy, good listeners, open-minded, non-reactive, and non-judgmental.
- Choose a place where you have sufficient privacy and a time where there are no distractions.
- Choose people whose loyalties are not divided and who will not feel the need to tell another friend or his or her spouse what you've shared.
- Keep in mind that therapists and clergy are sworn to maintain confidentiality so long as your stories don't involve doing potential harm to yourself or another person.

Freedom is an embodied experience that is not governed by your location or your circumstance. Nelson Mandela found his freedom during his 27-year period of incarceration. Freedom comes from within. As you begin to have embodied experiences of freedom, you can break the chains of your past and free yourself from cultural, social, psychological, and emotional tethers. Sharing our stories with each other is a beginning.

REST

Asana/posture

Practicing a side-lengthening pose like Reclined Half Moon Pose (Supta Ardha Chandrasana) supports lengthening the body which creates a sense of internal spaciousness. It allows your breath to deepen, expand, and circulate more fully from bottom to top, front to back, and side to side. When your breath is free to move without restriction, it helps release contraction in the nervous system and supports a feeling of expansiveness and freedom.

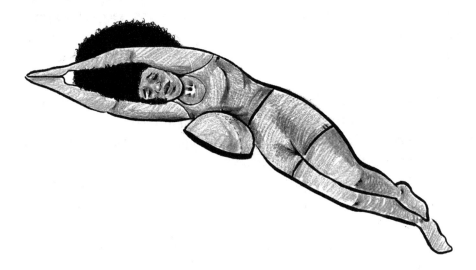

Place a bolster or a blanket roll horizontally in the middle of your mat. Sit with your right hip against the short end of your bolster or blanket roll; your legs are softly bent behind you with one leg on top of the other. Place a square folded blanket, block, or pillow between your knees if you like, and lean to the right. Place your right hand across the top of your bolster toward the far side of your mat and lower down over the bolster onto your right side. Once lowered onto the bolster, extend your right arm straight along the ground with your palm facing up and rest your head on your biceps. Extend your left arm straight up overhead with your palm facing the short edge of the mat. Lower your arm over your ear until both right and left palms touch. Feel the length in your left side body. Observe your breath and notice how it guides the movements of your spine as you lengthen and release. Relax your entire body and pay special attention to your neck and side body as the breath circulates from front to back and around your rib cage. When you are ready to switch sides, slowly turn your body face-down, pause, enjoy your breath, and then gently press your hands into the ground to rise up. Repeat on the other side. Hold on each side for two to ten minutes.

REFLECT

Affirmations

While in the posture, silently repeat to yourself three times, "Breathing in, I feel expansive... Breathing out, I feel spacious." On your fourth inhale, silently repeat, "Expansive." On your exhale, silently repeat, "Spacious." Continue that repetition—inhale "Expansive," exhale "Spacious"—for at least five more rounds. Rest on one side, focusing on your breath for as long as you are comfortable, then repeat on the other side. After repeating your affirmations on each side, when you are ready to come out of this pose, take two or three deep diaphragmatic breaths, tuck your chin into your chest, and gently press your hands into the floor to lift back up to sitting.

Feeling expansive and spacious in the body while repeating the phrases "I feel expansive" or "I feel spacious" plants seeds that can take root in the nervous system of the individual, releasing contraction and allowing the free flow of energy to be a felt experience. It supports a reduction in physical tension and rigid thinking, allowing for more openness, freedom, and resilience. It strengthens the ability to experience softening without fear of harm, a new experience for people who are chronically stressed or traumatized.

RENEW

Journal

In your journal, finish the sentence "I feel expansive and spacious when..."

_____

_____

_____

_____

_____

_____

_____

_____

_____

_____

_____

_____

_____

_____

_____

_____

_____

_____

Journal how this practice benefits you.

_____

_____

_____

_____

_____

_____

_____

_____

_____

_____

_____

_____

_____

_____

_____

_____

_____

_____

_____

_____

_____

_____

Chapter 6

SELF-WORTH

A T THE end of every Restorative Yoga class, I always ask participants to choose one word that describes what they are feeling. I do this to give them an opportunity to share their lived experience. It seals the practice and supports them in being able to identify their emotional state. The participants usually choose words like peaceful, calm, relaxed, open, free, joyful, inspired. At the end of one of the practices, I was taken aback when a woman new to me and new to yoga chose the word "shame." It was totally unexpected. Shame is a difficult emotion to feel and an even harder emotion to admit to feeling. I waited until everyone finished sharing and then asked her to say more about her experience of shame. She said during the practice she felt ashamed because of all of the years she had put herself last and hadn't take care of herself. She said she had not realized how painful that was until her experience in the class revealed to her that she had never felt worthy of her own care. She said becoming aware of how she had always neglected herself, never making her own needs a priority, was life-changing. I thought it was an astounding and deeply profound awareness. It left me wondering where the disconnection between self and care originates, because she is not alone in her self-neglect. This, by the way, was a highly accomplished, well-educated woman, happily married, successful in her career, and financially solvent. All of the social measures of someone who is regarded as having value. What was missing? Why didn't she feel worthy of her own care?

The value of your existence is baked into your consciousness, beginning in childhood. It is something you absorb without thinking. When reinforced, over time, these feelings are so ingrained they become part of your identity. Without any awareness of where you learn your sense of worth, you can adopt inflated feelings of worth and unwarranted feelings of worthlessness. You don't feel worthless because you are but because you've learned to think of yourself that way. So where do thoughts that lead to feelings of unworthiness originate?

There was a time in American history when Black people were not recognized by law as human beings but were regarded as property to be bought and sold as commodities. Enslaved Blacks could not legally marry, were barred from meeting together in groups, were prohibited from learning to read and write, and had no claim to their children who could be bought and sold on the whim of the plantation owners. Solomon Northrup in his memoire *Twelve Years a Slave*, originally published in 1853, gives a firsthand account of his experience as an enslaved man.

Northrup, whose father had been enslaved, was a free man living in upstate New York with his wife and children when he was kidnapped and sold into slavery. He details life on the various Southern plantations where he slaved, including describing the methods that were used for cultivating cotton and sugar cane, as well as the daily atrocities of torture and threat that all those who were enslaved endured. An example he shares is the daily amount of cotton those who slaved in the fields had to pick. The cruel catch was that they had to exceed their pick from the day before to avoid being whipped the following day. No matter how much cotton they picked, it was never enough. As an example he tells the story of Patsey who picked five hundred pounds of cotton each day, and was subjected to the inhumane punishment of being whipped for not doing more. To add insult to injury she was repeatedly sexually assaulted by the owner of the plantation who would beat her into submission if she resisted. On top of that Patsey was continually persecuted by the plantation owner's wife who accused her of seducing her husband. Who Patsey was, was never considered. No matter how much she did, it was never enough. No matter how much wrong was done to her, she was the one accused of wrongdoing. Her worth was based solely on how much and how hard she worked on behalf of the plantation owner and his family. Northrup also wrote about how the system of chattel slavery not only brutalized, traumatized, and diminished those who were enslaved, it brutalized the enslavers as well causing them to behave in monstrous ways. He wrote that because of the daily suffering they imposed, they eventually became desensitized to their own cruelty and brutality. They lost contact with the feeling of shame that prevents inhumane treatment.[1]

When you are culturally conditioned to put yourself last, it becomes habitual.

Without awareness of who you really are at your core, intrinsically worthy just because you exist, you learn to treat yourself as insignificant. Unacknowledged and unhealed trauma is passed on from one generation to the next, from those who were victimized to those who did the victimizing. The United States is a nation embedded in unacknowledged and unhealed race-based trauma. None of us, regardless of our ethnic or racial identity, have escaped the consequences of the cruel legacy that the system of chattel slavery imposed. We need to heal collectively.

Race-based traumatic stress injury can alter your perceptions of yourself and of your estimation of your value. What do you think of yourself? How do you evaluate your worth? Do you rely on the approval of others to affirm your worth or do you have an internal measure that you use to determine your value? We live in a culture that conditions you to evaluate your worth based on how hard you work, how much you produce, what you own, how you look, who you know, and how popular you are. The problem is that these culturally conditioned measures are not immutable and can suddenly change, making them unreliable reflections of your real value. When you rely on your looks, the number of friends or, in the era of social media, the number of Facebook, Twitter, or Instagram followers you have, when you rely on what you own, how much money you have, or what you've accomplished, you're basing your worth on something external. As long as you depend on external measures to validate your worth, you will never feel worthwhile. It is the inner experience of worthiness that we seek. Relying on external measures of success cannot help you access or sustain that inner experience. No person, possession, or accomplishment can make you feel worthy. In order to feel good about yourself, you have to be comfortable in your own skin. This is where yoga comes in.

THE PANCHAMAYA KOSHA MODEL

The panchamaya kosha model is based on philosophical teachings derived from an ancient Vedantic text called the Taittiriya Upanishad. It teaches that individuals are composed of five layers of being or sheaths, called koshas. The five layers of being are the physical body, the pranic or energy body, the mental/emotional body, the intellectual/intuitive body, and the bliss body. The physical body is called the anamaya kosha; the pranic or energy body is called the pranamaya kosha; the mental/emotional body is called the manomaya kosha; the intellectual/intuitive body is called the vijnanamaya kosha; and the bliss body is called the anandamaya kosha. Each layer of being is more subtle than the next. The panchamaya kosha model holds that the human system is interconnected and functions optimally when there is a state of dynamic balance and harmony between all five sheaths or layers of being.

The five koshas map the body from the unseen to the manifest. They are the veils that cloud our perception of our essential nature as already whole and complete. According to the text, it is avidya, ignorance of our core nature, that is the source of all suffering. Each individual is understood to be an aspect of all-pervading consciousness. The awareness of our true nature is covered by the five sheaths that obscure the knowledge of our actual identity. The true self, though intangible, is that aspect of being that remains constant, never changing. It is ultimately the recognition of and identification with that aspect of self, regardless of situation or circumstance, where our sense of worthiness resides. The panchamaya kosha model brings awareness to each dimension of our being, thereby facilitating the integration of each aspect, allowing you to become established in the seat of your essential nature as unchanging consciousness. As you become established in your identity as consciousness, you realize that you are more than your body, your breath, your emotions, your thoughts, or your personality. You are the consciousness that is experiencing all of that. You don't have to change what you are experiencing, you just have to learn that you are not the experience itself. You are the one observing the experience. It is your frame of mind that determines your reaction to the experience.[2]

KOSHAS

The koshas are not objects but forms that arise within your consciousness. They act in a hierarchical fashion—each layer more refined than the next, but each layer influencing those below it. Whatever is held in the bliss body, the most subtle and intangible of the five sheaths, will affect all the other koshas. Anandamaya kosha is foundational to health and wellbeing, which is why we want to cultivate a relationship with it. So we begin here. As above, so below.

ANANDAMAYA KOSHA (BLISS BODY)

There is something inside of us as human beings that wants to thrive and knows that life is worth living. Yoga teaches us that the bliss body, the most hidden part of us, and the one closest to our spiritual nature, is experienced as the deeply felt sense that to be alive is good and that, at the deepest level of being, worthiness is your birth right. It is more than a feeling; it is an inner knowing that your nature is free and that love is your foundation. Your bliss body is not dependent on what you are experiencing externally, or what your life circumstance is. It is the experience of unexplainable joy, vibrancy, and wellbeing. The bliss body abides as your base and shines through you. It is the awareness that the essential nature of life is beneficent. This loving support aids us in times of illness, grief, sorrow, and difficulty, and is very nourishing. It is a quality of deep appreciation for life. Yoga teaches us to continually cultivate conditions that enhance our sense of inner wellbeing regardless of external circumstance. Practices that support anandamaya kosha include meditation, gratitude practices, any creative activity that absorbs the ego so completely that only the activity is important, devotional practices (Bhakti yoga), or selfless service (Karma yoga).

VIJNANAMAYA KOSHA (WISDOM OR AWARENESS BODY)

More subtle than thought, there is an inner sense of knowing that is referred to as the intellect or wisdom body. It is awareness that shines in the light of consciousness and helps us understand our thinking mind. It is the knowing that is not dependent on direct experience, but is based on the ability to access and listen to a deep inner voice, sometimes called intuition. It is our body of insight. When you are absorbed in a creative project or solving a problem, you are accessing the wisdom body. The wisdom body is not dependent on the five senses for guidance. It is a sixth sense, the part of you that does not have to have a direct experience to know. It is the part of you that knows without seeing, hearing, tasting, touching, or smelling. Harriet Tubman is an example of this level of knowing. She was a woman born into slavery who fled to Philadelphia, Pennsylvania, from Maryland to escape bondage. Once there, she became an abolitionist. She returned to Maryland 13 times and rescued 70 people, some of them family, bringing them to freedom. She relied on her intuitive wisdom, and her connection and surrender to a higher power (Ishvara Pranidhana) to find safe passage. As we cultivate alert awareness, at some point the wisdom body becomes our primary teacher and we trade in learning from direct experience for wisdom. Practices that help develop this aspect of being include meditation, Restorative Yoga, mindfulness, contemplative practices, and self-study.

MANOMAYA KOSHA (MENTAL/EMOTIONAL BODY)

The mental/emotional body consists of our thoughts, emotions, perceptions, beliefs, opinions, assumptions, and memories. Emotions are the physiological responses to our thoughts. Thoughts and emotions affect how we respond to illness and injury, and can be a cause of stress, the root cause of all dis-ease. The thinking mind conceptualizes the world, relying on information and reasoning. It helps us make meaning out of the world we occupy. Our thoughts and emotions are influenced by culture, family, socialization, and past experiences. Subject to change, thoughts and emotions are not always reliable. Sometimes we think something is good for us when it is not, and sometimes we think something is bad for us when it is actually good for us. Some of our thoughts are self-generated and others are random, seeming to come out of nowhere. Some of our thoughts are conscious and some of our thoughts are stored in the unconscious. Unconscious thoughts are the lifelong mental habits and thought patterns, called samskaras, that influence and can distort our perceptions of reality. Practices that help focus the mind are appropriate for addressing issues of manomaya kosha and include setting intentions, meditation, and affirmations.

PRANAMAYA KOSHA (VITAL ENERGY BODY)

The vital energy body, or the life force, is the spark of life that lights up a room when a baby is born and the dimming of the light when life leaves the body. This is the energy that science cannot harness. You cannot see prana, but you can feel it. For example, during an asana (postural yoga) practice, you might feel a surge of heat ripple through your body. During meditation, you might experience feeling uplifted and inspired. In a quiet moment communing with nature, you might feel a deep sense of grounding and peace. When this happens, you are connecting to your energy body. Breath is a conduit for prana and aids in revitalization. Prana is everywhere. You can feel energy moving in nature, in the food you consume, in your surroundings, and you can feel energy emanating from one human being to another. Consider how you feel in the presence of scattered erratic energy, hostile energy, dull energy, or loving energy. Everyone emanates their own energetic state. Feeling vibrant, lethargic, and calm are all attributes of the energy body. Vitality waxes and wanes. Practices that are appropriate to address the pranamaya kosha include breath practices, restorative practices, and meditation practices that are calming to both mind and emotion and that support the efficient use of energy.

ANAMAYA KOSHA (PHYSICAL BODY)

This is the most tangible aspect of yourself and the most difficult to change. It is called the food body because it is a modification of what you eat and drink. It involves the musculoskeletal structure of the body, and your internal organs. Physical sensations such as pain and stiffness, relaxation and pleasure, ease and effort are experienced in the physical body. Consciously inhabiting your physical body will bring more presence and ease to your life. Instead of sensing your body from the outside in, you begin to cultivate interoceptive awareness and sense the physical body from the inside out. This awareness supports you in making choices that enhance health and wellbeing. Practices that support the anamaya kosha involve active and restorative asana practices to improve strength, stamina, balance and coordination, pranayama (breath practices), healthy diet, and sleep practices.

BECAUSE YOU'RE WORTH IT

Collectively, we have been working on undoing the cruel legacy of enslavement by advancing ourselves personally, educationally, politically, and professionally. We lovingly embrace our texturized hair, our beautiful and varied skin tones, the shape of our noses, our lips, and our bodies. We've made self-care our mantra and we engage in practices like yoga and meditation that have made us stronger than ever. But our work is not done. Not yet. There's still more to do. The work we have to do now is to transform the pain of racial wounding that we have embodied—the emotional wounds that have accumulated over generations that are buried deep inside of us. No one else can do this work for us. No amount of changing systems, laws, or other people can heal that pain. The pain that needs healing inside of us is the pain born of the wounds of being dehumanized, devalued, silenced, marginalized, excluded, tortured, sexually violated, murdered, and falsely accused; the pain that caused us and still causes us to question our worth, the pain that wonders, "Am I good enough?" "Am I smart enough?" "Do I still have to work twice as hard to get half as far?" "Am I doing something wrong?" When you adopt standards that condition you to think of your educational achievements, your personal and professional accomplishments, your wealth, your possessions, and how hard you work as measures of your value and your worth, you fail to see that you are worthy independent of these external measures of value.

When your basic needs for security are met, when you're making a little money, have a decent job and money in the bank, own your home, a car, maybe even a boat, you feel secure and you don't worry too much about the way-down deep-inside feelings that cause you to question your worth. You can distract yourself with indulgences that masquerade as self-care; going to the spa, the gym, the hairdresser, taking a vacation trip, binge-watching television—and high on the list for many is retail therapy. The problem is these are short-term remedies that cannot substitute for the deep work required to heal the wounds of race-related stress and trauma. They just mask the symptoms. They're also costly, and during a pandemic that requires physical distancing, an economic downturn that has cost people their jobs, closed businesses, and curtailed travel, attempting to soothe ourselves in these ways is no longer safe and, in some instances, no longer possible. Without your normal distractions, you may find yourself coming face to face with emotional pain that has been buried for centuries. Now is the time to acknowledge, address, and heal from that pain. Now is a time to go deeper into your real value as a human being who has worth, not because of how you look, what you do, how much you have, or where you live, but because of who you are at your core. Now is the time to love and value yourself for being who you are as your most deeply authentic self, not for living up to who others need you to be.

Self-worth and abundance go hand in hand. They are yoked. When you shift your focus from making everyone and everything else a priority to valuing yourself, you move from surviving to thriving. When you move from surviving to thriving, you prosper—we all do. When you value yourself, you no longer rely on external measures of self-worth such as how hard you work, how many degrees you have, how big your house is, how fancy your car is, or wearing designer clothes. When you believe in yourself, you feel worthy. Feeling worthy is not the same as feeling deserving of special treatment or privileges—that's called entitlement. No one is entitled, but all of us are worthy and deserving.

REST

Asana/posture

One of the negative outcomes of ethnic and race-based stress and trauma is the internalized belief that "I am not worthy" or "I'm not enough." These beliefs cause people who are subjected to this form of stress and trauma to spend a lifetime trying to prove their worth and working much harder than they would if they did not feel the burden of trying to prove themselves worthy. Supported wide-legged forward fold (Uppa Vishta Konansana) is calming and offers an experience of ease and comfort that you may not feel you deserve, but you do.

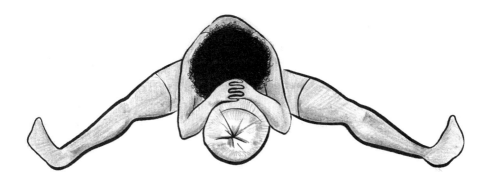

Sit on a blanket folded into a rectangular shape facing the long side of your mat and open your legs to a wide V position. Place the narrow end of the bolster between your legs. Fold forward from your groin, not your waist, and rest your forehead on the bolster. You should feel your legs and back body lengthening but not stretching. Use as much elevation on top of the bolster as you need to keep from over-stretching in this forward fold. You can do this by placing as many blocks as you need on top of the bolster for a head rest as you come into the forward fold. Your range of motion will determine how high your support needs to be. Rest your forehead on the support or turn your head to the side and rest your cheek on it. Use a square folded blanket or a rectangular folded blanket to cushion your head if you like. Rest your arms on either side of the bolster or drape them over the top. Hold this pose for five to ten minutes. When you are ready to come out of this pose, tuck your chin into your chest and lift your torso to an upright position, remove the bolster, place your hands behind your knees, and gently lift them until your feet are flat on your mat.

REFLECT

Affirmations

While in the posture, silently repeat to yourself three times, "Breathing in, I feel worthy... Breathing out, I feel deserving." On your fourth inhale, silently repeat, "Worthy." On your exhale, silently repeat, "Deserving." Continue that repetition—inhale "Worthy," exhale "Deserving"—for at least five more rounds. Rest in this posture, focusing on your breath for as long as you are comfortable. When you are ready to come out of this pose, take two or three deep diaphragmatic breaths, tuck your chin into your chest, and gently press your hands into the floor to lift back up to sitting.

Repeating the phrases "I feel worthy" and "I feel deserving" plants seeds that can take root in your consciousness and enable you to regard yourself as adequate and to regard your efforts as sufficient. Feeling adequate does not lead to complacency. It reduces self-doubt, increases self-confidence, and leads to greater efficacy.

RENEW

Journal

In your journal, finish the sentence "I feel worthy and deserving when..."

_____

_____

_____

_____

_____

_____

_____

_____

_____

_____

_____

_____

_____

_____

_____

_____

_____

_____

_____

_____

Journal how this practice benefits you.

_____

_____

_____

_____

_____

_____

_____

_____

_____

_____

_____

_____

_____

_____

_____

_____

_____

_____

_____

_____

_____

_____

Chapter 7

AUTHENTICITY

I WAS invited to be on a panel at a day-long yoga retreat in honor of Nelson Mandela Day by Yoga in Colour, a group of South African yogis dedicated to supporting inclusivity, diversity, empowerment, and healing within the broader yoga community. Two things that stood out for me in the discussion about culturally informed yoga practices involved authenticity and identity. The first was that Black South Africans described feeling like imposters in predominantly White yoga spaces, as if they did not belong, unless they could prove their worth by demonstrating how well they could perform when doing the yoga postures. The other was that, in spite of or maybe because of South African apartheid, Black South Africans have remained connected to their indigenous roots, an important aspect of identity and a source of cultural pride and strength.

One of the deepest wounds of African Americans is the erasure of African ancestral and cultural roots along with individual identity. It began during the Trans-Atlantic slave trade. Kidnapped from their homeland, shackled together in the hull of slave ships, men and women from various African nations and cultures, with different customs, languages, and religions, were lumped into one category. Deprived of their families, their homes, their hopes and dreams, even their own names, "slave" became their new identity. Slavery in America involved stripping human beings of their individual identity and turning them into property. From its inception, enslavement in the United States was conditioned on the basis of skin color alone. Black became synonymous with slave, and skin color, not culture, eventually became and continues to be the most important aspect of American identity.

Your individual identity is how you view yourself as unique from others. Cultural identity is learned and passed on from one generation to the next.

It includes the beliefs, value systems, social structures, support networks, history, food, religion, language, and customs that bind a community of people together. Being ripped from one's homeland, robbed of one's culture, separated from one's family, deprived of one's name and all that is familiar is traumatic. Unprocessed trauma is retained in the body and passed on from one generation to the next. When we attempt to override it with spiritual bypassing or magical thinking or compartmentalizing, or ignoring, we deny ourselves the gift of renewal. We can avoid all of this by first looking within to heal our wounds.

FIRST LOOK WITHIN

Trauma often leads people to become seekers as a way to come to terms with or understand themselves at deeper levels beyond culture, race, and ethnicity. Many trauma survivors are drawn to yoga practices intuitively, without realizing that it is more than just a physical practice. It is actually a practice that offers opportunities for self-discovery that can provide new ways of knowing yourself. Yoga prepares you for the inner journey and helps you cultivate an inner-oriented perspective that leads to transformation and growth. Paramahansa Yogananda taught that it is through your yoga practices that you can find meaning, authenticity, and a personal experience of truth that you are more than your individual, socially and culturally conditioned identities. He taught that within each of us is a steady place that is not fraudulent. It cannot be located or defined, but it is a place of truth that can be experienced. It is a place of safety, comfort, and wellbeing that permeates all aspects of our being. It is where we find solace and peacefulness, reassuring us that all is well regardless of external events or circumstances. It is the place where love finds its way into your heart, where joy and bliss erupt spontaneously for no apparent reason, and where you experience the peace that passes understanding. In this place, you can access your creativity and potential. In this place, you can transform and rise like the Egyptian Phoenix from the ashes of loss and despair. This aspect of self is whole and complete, and can never be damaged or broken. It is the most subtle aspect of your being, where the truth of your identity resides.

If you are someone who is on a path of self-discovery, you will discover that periodically, throughout your lifetime, you will feel the urge to grow beyond the person you've been socialized to be. You will feel an urge to explore the hidden parts of yourself, the parts of yourself that you yearn to be. If you choose the path of self-discovery, you will soon learn that it requires courage to step into your truth and authenticity because exploring the unknown requires radical openness, which requires a willingness to step into your vulnerability. There is a threat to knowing the unknown about yourself because it can be strange, foreign, and in some cases unwanted. On the journey to self-discovery, you risk profound change and you risk becoming someone who is not the same as you thought you were. Radical openness involves sitting with the discomfort of that which might be true, including ways that you may have neglected yourself and ways that you may have harmed others. We are attached to our own sense of personal goodness which interferes with our ability to discover anything that challenges that notion of self. Our perceptions of self are filtered through the cultural norms we have been taught and through our own lived experience. We do not always see as clearly as we think we do, but through a filmy layer of our conditioning and past experiences. This results in faulty perceptions or incorrect understanding. The Yoga Sutra calls these misapprehensions avidya. But Patanjali's Sutra tells us that there is a deeper level of perception that is not obscured by avidya. Yoga aims to remove our blinders so that we can become more aware and open to the unknown aspects of ourselves so that we can see with more clarity.

THE JOURNEY TO SELF-DISCOVERY

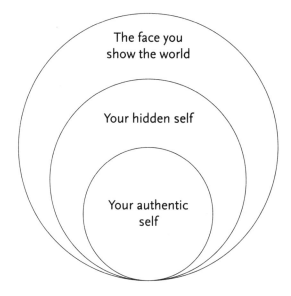

The face you
show the world

Your hidden self

Your authentic
self

YOU ALREADY ARE WHO YOU'RE TRYING TO BECOME

Individual, cultural, racial, ethnic, and gender identity are social constructs that are conditioned and changeable. You are more than that. A remnant of race-based traumatic stress that clouds perception is called high-effort coping. It is a behavioral style that people who are locked out of opportunities and access to resources engage in as a means of gaining access and to prove their worth. High-effort coping is a way of functioning based on the belief that in order to measure up, you have to make a two-hundred-percent effort in all that you do. Giving a two-hundred-percent effort to endeavors is a way of functioning that makes rest and relaxation foreign because you think that the harder you try, and the more effort you make, the better you are doing. This is an adaptive response to being denied equal access to the rights of full citizenship, fueled by the belief that by making extraordinary efforts, all obstacles to justice, representation, and equity can be overcome. Balancing out this commitment to making extraordinary efforts requires recognizing that trying your hardest is not the same as doing your best. What if it turns out that doing your best is good enough? What if, instead of aspiring to do more and be more, as was required during enslavement, you aspired to be your best self and operate from that frame of reference?

Being referred to as underserved, marginalized, underprivileged, and at risk reinforces deficiencies and exacerbates feelings of worthlessness. The most damaging impact of these labels is the internalization of low self-esteem and the belief that in some way you are limited in your potential, which makes you doubt your accomplishments and abilities, and leaves you feeling like an imposter or a fraud. But here's the truth. We live in a world of infinite possibility and each of us has unlimited potential. The trick is learning how to access your possibilities and actualize your potential. Accessing your possibilities and actualizing your potential cannot be done by trying to live up to, or down to, others' expectations of you. You have capacities that are unique to you and you alone. You have your own optimal blueprint, and within that blueprint are contained your unique possibilities. Another way of thinking about this is to consider that a seed holds within it the potential to become what it is. It cannot be anything else. For example, the seed of a sunflower can only manifest as a sunflower. Operating within its own blueprint, it will never become a violet. It can only be a sunflower no matter how much it tries to be something else. Trying to fit a mold that is not of your making is the same as trying to become someone you're not. You cannot fulfill someone else's potential, no matter how hard you try. This does not mean you shouldn't aspire to grow. It does mean you should aspire to be clear that the answers to who you are lie deep within your own being, not in someone else's version of who they think you should be. There's an old saying that applies here: "What you think of me is none of my business."

Trying to be someone you're not is an energy drain and tends to be a waste of time. We tend to do our best at what we do the best. The most successful people in the world know this. They focus on and build on their strengths instead of trying to improve on their limitations and deficiencies. How do you know what you do best? You know by paying attention to what you truly love, what comes easiest to you, and what you're naturally good at. This is not necessarily an easy path, especially when there are barriers in place to hold you back, but following this path is how we grow and remain strong even in the face of adversity. Your authentic self is synonymous with your best self. You and your unique gifts are irreplaceable. The planet needs a diversity of talents and abilities if we are to succeed as individuals, families, communities, and nations. The world needs you to be who you are and to express your unique gifts and talents.

You have to align with the best in you. If your ultimate goal is to be your authentic self, your immediate goal is to get on the path that will lead you there. To do that, you have to line up with what you love and let your passion lead you, even when you'd rather not. Without passion for doing something, you'll never be successful, because you won't be able to sustain the energy necessary to continue on when you are faced with the inevitable challenges that will come your way. Fulfilling your potential requires going beyond the goal of making money. It takes everything you have to give: all your talent, energy, focus, commitment, and all your love, but the rewards are worth it. You create purpose and meaning in your life when you consciously choose on behalf of what your purpose is. What you love and what's most important to you contain clues to your purpose. We actually become what we love.

What you dislike doing most is probably not what you are best suited for, and it is a waste of time trying to get better at something that doesn't suit you. Why not use your energy getting better at something you enjoy, something you're already good at, something you really love? Pelé, the famed Brazilian soccer player, is an example. In defiance of his coaches, he stopped trying to play soccer in the European style and began to play soccer by embracing his

African Brazilian roots. He was a natural when it came to the ginga, a special rhythmic way of moving that is regarded as the soul of Brazilian football. This style of play was denigrated by Europeans as primitive and forbidden by his coaches. Pelé tried his hardest to conform but proved to be mediocre playing in the European style. Eventually, he found the courage to honor his roots. Once he did, his innate gifts and talents emerged, and he discovered who he really was and what he was capable of doing on the soccer field. In 1958, Pelé helped Brazil win its first World Cup. There is nothing more powerful than tapping into who you already are and building on that.

It is by doing what you love and what you are good at that you serve the greater good. When you forget about what people will think of you and instead concern yourself with how you can be most helpful to them, you are engaged in what the Bhagavad Gita calls skill in action. The Gita tells us that when we engage in the yoga of wisdom and accept reality as it is, not as we want it to be, when we selflessly serve others by doing what we do simply for the sake of it and for the joy of doing it, and when we surrender and let go of any expected or hoped-for outcome and accept what life has to offer and is asking of us, we are engaged in right action. We are operating from our authentic self.

We serve others best when we commit to looking for and focusing on our innate inner talents and then using those abilities to be the best for the world. When you make doing what you love and what you're good at your focus, you have a greater chance of getting better at it, eventually gaining mastery of it, and of being truly successful. When you make doing something that helps other people your focus, it gives you a reason to get up in the morning and motivates you to keep going even when things are tough.

When we focus on our innate gifts and talents, those things that come most naturally and easiest to us, we support growth. Even when we are faced with obstacles that seem insurmountable, when we are in alignment with our natural abilities, and when we are in touch with our authenticity, we have the energy and the motivation to keep going. In spite of the obstacles you are faced with, you refuse to accept the limitations others try to place on you, and you begin to see every obstacle as just another opportunity. Obstacles can be overcome by committing to relentlessly follow your heart's deepest desires, no matter who or what opposes you. By living life authentically and facing your fears head on, you can transform stressful and traumatic events, and you can grow from the hardships and heartache they bring.

Focusing on your strengths supports proficiency and the ability to function with ease. It doesn't mean that you don't work hard and make the necessary efforts to achieve your goals or to function with intention and purpose. But to function with ease means to use your energy wisely. We do not have unlimited energy, and using it wisely requires self-awareness and self-care practices so that we are not depleted.

REST

Asana/posture

A supported Downward-Facing Corpse Pose (Savasana) is a restful pose that rejuvenates. This resting pose offers an experience of resting in stillness in a way that can support relaxation and ease, balancing out effort. You already are who you're trying to become.

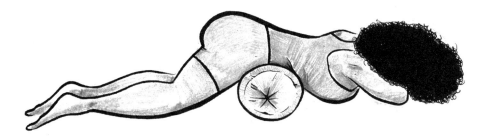

Place a bolster, rectangular folded blanket, or rolled blanket horizontally across the middle of your mat. Facing the top end of your mat, kneel at the bolster or blanket. Position your hips at the bolster or blanket and lay your torso across the top so that your hips are raised on it. Extend your arms forward with bent elbows and place one hand on top of the other, creating a cushion for your head. Lower your forehead onto your hands or turn your head to one side, resting on your cheek. Let your legs and feet relax, and let your heels fan out toward the outer edges of your mat while your toes turn in. Hold this pose for five to 20 minutes. Focus on your breath. When you are ready to come out of this pose, press your hands into the floor and, with your chin tucked, lift yourself back off the bolster or blanket, and come into child's pose with your arms draped horizontally over the bolster. Hold here for at least five full diaphragmatic breaths and then lift up to sitting.

REFLECT

Affirmations

While in the posture, silently repeat to yourself three times, "Breathing in, I feel authentic... Breathing out, I feel at ease." On your fourth inhale, silently repeat, "Authentic." On your exhale, silently repeat, "Ease." Continue that repetition—inhale "Authentic," exhale "Ease"—for at least five more rounds. Rest in this posture, focusing on your breath, for as long as you are comfortable. When you are ready to come out of this pose, take two or three deep diaphragmatic breaths, tuck your chin into your chest, and gently press your hands into the floor to lift back up to sitting.

Repeating the phrases "I feel authentic" and "I feel at ease" plants seeds that give permission to find the ease and relaxation that balance extraordinary effort. All effort does not have to be hard work. It supports the recognition that working harder and doing one's best are not the same. It makes the notion of doing something with ease attractive and removes the fear of being considered a malingerer if one is not working to prove one's value. Supported Downward-Facing Savasana is a comforting, calming pose that leads to an overall sense of wellbeing. Deep belly, or diaphragmatic, breathing comes naturally in this pose, creating a sense of peace. Peacefulness is an inner state of being. Feeling peaceful is an unfamiliar feeling for people who are chronically stressed or traumatized. The ability to experience feeling at ease and not on high alert while being still is new and comforting.

RENEW

Journal

In your journal, finish the sentence "I feel authentic and at ease when…"

_____

_____

_____

_____

_____

_____

_____

_____

_____

_____

_____

_____

_____

_____

_____

_____

_____

_____

_____

_____

_____

_____

Journal how this practice benefits you.

_____

_____

_____

_____

_____

_____

_____

_____

_____

_____

_____

_____

_____

_____

_____

_____

_____

_____

_____

_____

_____

Chapter 8

LOVE

IN THE opening scene of Toni Morrison's opera *Margaret Garner*, the true story of an enslaved woman on a Kentucky plantation who attempted to escape to begin a new life, a family in the plantation slave quarters is celebrating the birth of their baby. Both mother and father are filled with love, joy, and hope for the possibility of a better future for their child. Knowing the horrors and heartbreak of enslavement, the grandmother warns them, "Don't love that baby too much." Her warning to withhold love was a warning born of her experience of the painful loss of loved ones sold as property to other plantations, never to be seen again, and the pain of helplessness and humiliation experienced in the face of the daily brutality she and others endured. Her warning was a defense to protect the heart, a seed planted in our collective consciousness that has been passed down through the ages, causing many of us to guard our hearts from the unbearable emotional pain and suffering that enslavement imposed.

The fear of loving too much is an adaptive response to the cruel legacy of chattel slavery and a residual of race-based stress and trauma. Denying the depth of one's love is a defense erected to protect against a painful past of separation from loved ones and the heartbreak that enslaved people had to endure. But the truth is, withholding love does not protect us. You can survive without love, but you cannot thrive without it. Love is the deepest longing of your heart. It is your nature. It is who you are.

YOU ARE LOVE

"I love you, Mommy. You are love." When my five-year-old son said this to me, I was astounded. He recognized something about who I was that until that moment I had not considered. I thought of love as something you feel, something you give, something you receive, or something you withhold, not who you actually are. I thought of love as something external to me, not something that is me. "You are love" is a concept the mystics taught, not something I expected to hear from a five-year-old child. It made me think of all the years I'd spent longing for, looking for, and waiting for love. I was searching for something on the outside that would make me feel good on the inside, without realizing that something external could never make me feel good internally. I was searching for something that was hiding in plain sight. I was just looking in the wrong place.

My son's sweet remarks made me yearn to have an inner experience of me *as* love. Sometimes it's hard to remember that we are the embodiment of love, that the purpose of life is spiritual growth, that our calling is to recreate a world with more love and compassion in it, and to establish a norm of love in all of our interactions with others, beginning with ourselves. Recognizing yourself *as* love is the supreme act of self-love.

LOVE YOURSELF

The practice of self-love is important because no one can love you better than you can love yourself—nor can you love anyone else better than you can love yourself. Loving others more than you love yourself is an energy drain that leads to great disappointment, bitterness, anger, and resentment. Looking for love from others drains them and leaves you feeling deprived and empty like a bottomless pit. Learning to love yourself and, even better, to recognize yourself *as* love itself leads to fulfillment. This is not to say that we do not need others. We do. We long to live in community and in right relationship. But a prerequisite to loving community and right relationship is the ability to take good care of yourself. Taking good care of yourself is a necessary step to being able to serve others lovingly. Many of us learn to equate self-love with vanity and selfishness. Actually, the more loving, kind, generous, and patient you are with yourself, the more these qualities will manifest *as* you and in your relationships with others. Self-love has the power to enhance relationships even if only one person in the relationship practices it. It is transformational. There are five aspects of self-love that if practiced will open your heart to loving yourself, to loving your life, and to recognizing that indeed you are the embodiment of love itself.

Kindness is first. In order to develop a loving relationship with ourselves, we must be committed to treating ourselves with loving kindness in thought, word, and deed. It means we must make peace with and affirm ourselves. We must refrain from thinking of ourselves negatively, calling ourselves names in anger, or engaging in behavior that is in any way harmful to us. We must be radically affirmative in our relationship to ourselves.

Authenticity is the second aspect of self-love. We must be open to the truth of our being. We must be willing to be who we are. This is what is meant by the saying "To thine own self be true." Each one of us has been given special gifts and talents to fulfill our purpose. To ignore, reject, or misuse these innate abilities is an act of self-rejection and undermines our sense of self-worth and our ability to be in right relationship with others. Love yourself for who you actually are, not for who you think someone expects you to be. It is better to strive toward being who you are than to excel at being someone you are not. March to the beat of your own drum.

Gratitude is the third aspect of self-love. It is important to practice appreciating what you have, and who you are. Many of us spend far too much time focusing on what we wish we had, or what we don't have, which leads to deep inner suffering. We think that having what we don't have will alleviate our suffering. Actually, it is our focus on what we don't have, not the absence of something, that leads to our suffering. As long as you are comparing yourself with others as being better or worse than you, you will suffer, and you will deprive yourself of peacefulness and contentment in your life.

Balance is the fourth aspect of self-love that we need to develop. We need to be able to flow comfortably between giving and receiving. Some people find it easier to give, while others find it easier to receive. If giving comes more naturally to you, you will eventually have a need to receive. If receiving comes more naturally to you, you will eventually have a desire to give. We need to be able to both give and receive to balance our personalities.

Forgiveness is the fifth aspect of self-love. Forgiving ourselves for our mistakes is an act of self-love that requires letting go of shame, blame, criticism, and self-accusation. There are four steps to self-forgiveness. Identify what you think you've done wrong. Let yourself feel the remorse associated with what you've done. Promise not to do it again and keep the promise. Then let it go.

LOVE YOUR LIFE

Any one of these five aspects, if practiced consistently and with patience, will inevitably lead to self-love, the foundation of loving your life. But to accomplish this, you have to walk the path of self-love with dedication. It is difficult to remain on a path that doesn't feel natural so here is a practice that might assist you. There is a center in the body where love, compassion, and trust reside. It is the spiritual heart center. Your spiritual heart center lies just behind the breastbone. Close your eyes and be aware of your heart as a space. Let your attention rest easily there. Breathe gently and sense your breath going gently into your heart center. As you do this, ask your heart to speak to you, and for the next few minutes just rest in silence and listen. Whatever message your heart has for you, know that it is beneficial. When you love yourself, you love your life.

Self-love is the willingness to cherish yourself for who you are, not for who someone else needs you to be. Without self-love, it is impossible to love your life or to love others, yet self-love is not traditionally thought of as being the foundation for loving your life. Self-love is not self-indulgence, but love of self that demonstrates that we regard ourselves as worthy. When we regard ourselves as worthy, we treat ourselves accordingly in thought, word, and deed. Self-love comes from the heart and results in an open heart that allows you to experience and express the love you actually are. Loving your life is a tall order to fill. Knowing how can be a challenge. Like anything that seems too big to manage, reducing it into bite-size pieces helps.

STOP, LOOK, LISTEN TO YOUR HEART

In order to love, we must approach life with an open heart. In order to remain open-hearted, we need to feel psychologically and emotionally safe. The built-in intelligence of the heart causes it to contract and protect itself if it does not feel safe. So how do we create emotional and psychological safety as we invite our hearts to remain open even in the face of great challenge, including the heartbreak of racial injustice and violence?

What comes to mind is the fictional story of Harry, a financially successful businessman, who was more concerned with the bottom line of his company than he was with treating his employees with care and respect. When Harry suffers a heart attack and is in the liminal state between life and death, an angel instructs him to follow five principles of caring for and about others. If he agrees to follow these principles, he will be given a second chance at life. Though skeptical and somewhat resistant, in order to gain that second chance he accepts the challenge. Once he accepts the challenge, he regains consciousness and even before he leaves the hospital begins to practice the five principles of love and caring toward others that the angel taught him.[1] But the principles Harry learned from the angel can also be used to relate to yourself. Just imagine how life might change for you and those around you if you applied these five principles of emotional and psychological safety to your own internal dialogue…if you managed yourself from your heart.

Hear and understand me. Just as others need to feel heard and understood, you need to feel heard and understood too. It starts with you. When you listen to yourself with an attitude of understanding, you hear yourself more clearly and you are more likely to feel understood and listened to by others.

Even if you disagree with me, please don't make me wrong. No one likes to be invalidated or have his or her worth questioned, which is what happens when you criticize someone for being wrong. They usually become defensive and communication stops. The same thing happens when you treat yourself this way. How often do you get into arguments with yourself about what you're thinking, feeling, or doing? What kind of inner turmoil do you think you create for yourself when you disagree with yourself and tell yourself how wrong you are? Notice when you do this how you shut down.

Acknowledge the greatness within me. Everyone has the potential to grow and responds positively to someone who addresses his or her potential greatness. When you acknowledge your own potential for growth and greatness, you become your own best friend. You become your own cheerleader and you enhance your capacity for growth and greatness.

Remember to look for my loving intentions. Give yourself the benefit of the doubt that your intention is to make things better. This even applies when you make a mistake. When you make mistakes or come up with an idea that others may not fully understand or appreciate, are you willing to give yourself the benefit of the doubt and trust that your intention really is to make things better?

Tell yourself the truth with compassion. Are you caring and respectful when you talk to yourself? Do you apply the principles of right speech to your internal dialogue about yourself? Before criticizing, shaming, or blaming yourself, do you ask yourself these three questions: Is it true? Is it necessary? Is it kind?[2]

Make a commitment to become an emotionally and psychologically safe person. Apply these principles to yourself and applying them to others will become second nature. You'll like yourself a lot more and others will like you more too.

RECEIVING LOVE

When you have been exposed to ongoing racial stress and trauma and have learned to protect your heart, it can be difficult to openly receive love. When you feel obliged to be strong no matter what—to suppress displays of emotion, to be stoic in the face of physical and emotional pain, to be fiercely independent, not needing anyone, rarely if ever asking for help, to succeed no matter what the obstacles or cost to your health or wellbeing, and to put others' needs ahead of your own—you need to feel loved and cared for. But as much as we need to be loved, due to past unhealed trauma, we erect walls to protect ourselves from feeling vulnerable. Think about the times you automatically dismiss a compliment, refuse support when it's offered, find ways to emotionally distance yourself from someone trying to be close, deflect attention away from yourself, or start an argument with someone trying to show you love and affection. Notice what happens when someone treats you in a loving way—let's say something as simple as telling you, "You look great." Can you receive the compliment? Are you able to say, "Thank you"? Or do you contract and withdraw and say something like, "Well, I've seen better days." Minimizing what the other person says keeps the compliment from getting all the way in and cracking open your defenses.

Sometimes we distract ourselves from receiving love by trying to feign indifference, as if we don't care. We might dull our senses with comfort food, alcohol, gambling, drugs (illegal and prescription), television, work, and our electronic devices. But why? If love is our essence, why do we protect ourselves from it? For those who have suffered race-based stress and trauma, receiving love can be much more of a challenge than giving it. One of the reasons is that to receive love, you have to make yourself vulnerable. Being vulnerable opens you up to those parts of yourself that you may have learned to keep hidden such as feeling unworthy and undeserving, or the part of you that learned that it's selfish to receive love, or the part of you that feels weak in your vulnerability. Letting love in, receiving love, opens you to all of the feelings hidden behind your firewall of protection. As much as you may want to receive love, an aversion to exposing these hidden parts of yourself can cause you to keep others from getting too close to you.

But numbing yourself to the discomfort of your vulnerability does more than dull the sting of unpleasant emotions. It keeps you from receiving love. You actually put yourself at a disadvantage by robbing yourself of the ability to ask for and receive the love and support you need. Ironically, by avoiding your vulnerability, you actually deprive yourself of the protection that comes from acknowledging it. In reality, we are all vulnerable and knowing that helps us get our needs met and helps keep us out of harm's way. Rather than hiding behind a wall of protection, increase your capacity to receive love. Find the courage to step into your vulnerability.

Vulnerability is not a sign of weakness. Admitting to and sharing your most tender parts—what you don't know, what you're not good at, what scares you, what hurts you—as well as your most cherished dreams and aspirations, requires deep inner strength. We fear being vulnerable because we fear being hurt, let down, disappointed, mocked, or rejected. Ultimately, nothing can protect you from the vulnerability of human life. When you stop avoiding your own vulnerability, you risk hurt and disappointment, but you receive the gifts that flow forth from a place of open-heartedness—kindness, forgiveness, love, generosity, empathy, and support.

REST

Asana/posture

Yoga invites us into intimacy with ourselves and with each other. A supported back bend, bridge pose (Setu Bandha Sarvangasana) is heart-opening. It may seem counter-intuitive, but opening your heart, even when it's aching, is healing. An open heart is a courageous heart. It is not afraid to love. Love is what heals our wounded hearts. An open heart is able to express itself in harmony with whatever is happening in the moment. It cries when it's sad, rages when it's mad, finds courage when it's afraid, and loves from its depth. Opening your heart to love opens your heart to compassion for yourself and for others. Supported back bending is a heart-opening practice that allows your heart to open to both giving and receiving love.

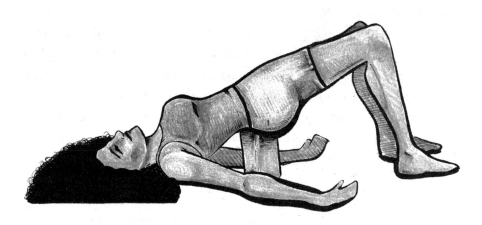

Lie down on your mat. Bend your knees with your feet flat on the mat about hip distance apart and about six inches from your buttocks. Lift your hips, and place a block, bolster, or folded blanket under your hips. Choose the height that feels best under your lower back. Remember that comfort, not intensity, is key. Lower your hips onto the prop you have chosen. Relax with your arms extended along the sides of your body and your palms facing up, or in cactus position. If you choose cactus position, lift your arms out to the sides of your body in the shape of a "T" at shoulder height. Bend your elbows to 90 degrees. Keep your upper arms horizontal and bend your forearms back behind you until the backs of your hands are flat on the ground. Focus your awareness on your breath. Remain in this pose for a minimum of three minutes to a maximum of ten minutes. When you are ready, lift your hips, remove the prop, and lower yourself to the floor. Roll onto your right side, coming into fetal position, and rest here for five to ten full breaths. Tuck your chin into your chest and use the strength in your arms to lift up to sitting, with your head following last.

This is not recommended for women who are more than three months pregnant.

REFLECT

Affirmations

While in the posture, silently repeat to yourself three times, "Breathing in, I feel open... Breathing out, I feel love." On your fourth inhale, silently repeat, "Open." On your exhale, silently repeat, "Love." Continue that repetition—inhale "Open," exhale "Love"—for at least five more rounds. Rest in this posture, focusing on your breath for as long as you are comfortable. When you are ready to come out of this pose, take two or three deep diaphragmatic breaths, remove the block from under your hips, roll to your right side, and come into fetal position. Rest here before tucking your chin into your chest, and gently pressing your hands into the floor to lift back up to sitting. Repeating the phrases "I feel open" and "I feel love" plants seeds that support a feeling of safety in one's vulnerability.

RENEW

Journal

In your journal, finish the sentence "I feel open and loving when..."

_____

_____

_____

_____

_____

_____

_____

_____

_____

_____

_____

_____

_____

_____

_____

_____

_____

_____

_____

Journal how this practice benefits you.

_____

_____

_____

_____

_____

_____

_____

_____

_____

_____

_____

_____

_____

_____

_____

_____

_____

_____

_____

_____

_____

_____

Chapter 9

PATIENCE

T HERE ONCE was a wise and humble man who had the most extraordinary gift. He could relate to anyone and got along with everyone. He never argued with friends, family, coworkers, or even strangers. His marriage was happy, and his children were well behaved, respectful, kind, and polite. He enjoyed remarkable harmony inside and outside of his home. News of this amazing man traveled to the Emperor of the land who was so intrigued by the man's reputation that he ordered him to come to the palace in order to meet him in person. After meeting with him, the Emperor ordered the man, by royal proclamation, to write a ten-thousand-word document describing how everyone in the empire could create loving, peaceful relationships as he had done. The man was then sent off to write. Five days later he returned to the palace with a heavy scroll that was immediately taken to the great hall and rolled out across a huge table. The Emperor's court stood silently by as the Emperor began to read the scroll. In just a few minutes, much to everyone's delight, he nodded his approval. The man had written ten thousand words as the Emperor requested—but it was the same word written over and over and over again: Patience, Patience, Patience.

PATIENCE IS LOVING

The foundation of patience is love. Every loving heart overflows with it. Patience is the way a mother shows her love to a toddler having a meltdown, or the love a husband shows his wife when she's running late, or the love a son shows his mother learning to use the latest technological gadget. Love and patience go together like hand-in-glove. It is the loving response to frustration. Have you ever watched a small child trying to pour a glass of milk with unsteady hands? Can you wait to see if he actually needs your help to avoid a spill before you grab the milk carton and pour it yourself? If your wife (husband) is driving to a destination and appears to be lost, can you wait to see if she (he) asks for your help before you offer a suggestion? How much frustration can you tolerate before you intervene with a solution to someone else's problem? Patience makes room for the power of love to work on a troubled relationship. It empowers love to care for a troubled child, and empowers us to take care of ourselves when we are troubled. It helps us realize that we do have time to set aside 20 minutes a day for our own wellbeing, even if we tell ourselves we don't. Exercising patience allows you to share your perspective with those who may see things differently from you with compassion and respect, in a mentoring rather than a judgmental or scolding way. The ability to remain open to love in every moment requires patience. Just when you think you have come to the end of your rope and your patience has run out, love empowers you to endure just a little bit longer.

PATIENCE EMPOWERS

Patience is the ability to experience frustration, difficulty, or inconvenience with equanimity. It is not just a matter of waiting; it is also a matter of timing. It is the ability to discern the right time to act, for the right reasons, in the right way. Learning patience takes time and practice. It is measured by the capacity to tolerate uncertainty while waiting for an opportunity or a desired outcome; waiting for the relationship you long for to manifest, waiting to hear the outcome of an important job interview, for an injury to heal, or an illness to abate. We wait patiently not for the sake of endurance, and not passively without doing what we can, but in the recognition that we all have the ability to tolerate a frustration, an unpleasant experience, an inconvenience, or uncertainty until it passes.

Patience is a superpower that requires strength and perseverance. It is the driver that increases our capacity to look forward to a brighter future with an open heart while we fight for reforms that provide equitable treatment, justice, and opportunity for all. It inspires us to keep pushing on to achieve our goals even when we face obstacles or delays. Being patient is not the same as being passive. Passivity is the unwillingness or inability to act, because we would rather not rock the boat or stir the pot. It lacks intention, courage, and discipline. It is an expression of indifference, of not caring, and is actually the withholding of love. It is a sign of a lack of interest or concern. Patience on the other hand is engaged, intentional, disciplined, and compassionate.

PATIENCE IS WISE

There is a limitless presence within you, an intelligence beyond the thinking mind, a sense of knowing that, if followed, leads you to your soul's purpose. Some call it our North Star. It is your inner guide, the part of you that is unchanging, that you can depend on no matter what else is going on around you. Exercising patience slows you down long enough to pause and take a deep breath so you can listen to your intuitive guidance, the wisdom that leads you to your soul's purpose, and gets you back on track whenever you lose your way. When you listen to your intuitive intelligence and operate from a place of insight and wisdom, you become discerning and you're able to step into your full power and potential. You learn not to be afraid of following your passion because you notice that when you do, a series of events that encourage you to keep going forward will show up in your life. Practicing patience teaches you to wait for answers to emerge from that place of deep inner knowing before you act. "Patience is the companion of wisdom."[1]

PATIENCE IS TIMELESS

Your experience of time is subjective and culturally determined, influencing your relationship to patience. In other words, time is not an absolute. Americans live in a fast-paced culture that expects instant gratification, and some of us think and act as if even that takes too long. The more you can accomplish in the shortest amount of time is considered a measure of success. This cultural norm plays a role in how we think, feel, and behave. It's easy to be patient when things are going well, but can you be patient when you're frustrated or suffering? When things don't go your way, when you have to wait for someone or something, or when you don't get the outcome you hope for, do you become impatient? Impatience is based on a cultural belief that time itself is finite and divided into days, weeks, hours, months, seconds, and years. But the division of time into linear measurements reflects how we perceive change, not how things really are. Thinking that time is finite causes us to believe that time can run out. That belief leads us to behave as if we have to beat the clock, that time is of the essence, that we have to hurry up, get things done, and cram everything in; otherwise, we are seen as wasting time. This way of thinking is stressful. The physicists tell us that time is actually eternal, that it never runs out. When we embody and metabolize the fact that time is infinite, we begin to recognize that we have all the time in the world and we reduce our stress.

Awareness is what creates the way you experience time. Restorative Yoga and meditation practices offer the experience of timelessness. Your awareness of timelessness contributes to a significant shift in your consciousness that translates into a sense of ease that supports you in being patient with yourself and others. The experience of patience is actually the embodiment of time-lessness. You begin to recognize that being impatient does not change how quickly something gets done; it just stresses you out. You begin to realize that being impatient does not rush an outcome. It simply frustrates you because you have not yet achieved a desired goal. Impatience is actually a sign that you feel helpless and powerless. You're not. Rather than pushing or rushing to get an outcome, yoga teaches you that putting all you have into your actions, doing your best to accomplish a task, and then releasing attachment to an outcome is your practice. This is where your power resides. This attitude helps you cultivate patience. But it requires a willingness to sit in the fire of your own impatience without trying to force an outcome while you wait for a result.

I participated in a year-long meditation training that required, among other things, meditating for 20 minutes twice each day. It was during a period in my life when I felt overwhelmed, given my responsibilities as a wife, a mother, a caretaker of an aging parent, and as a professional. Being still was not something I had practiced. Initially, sitting in stillness felt like torture to me and made me feel as if I wanted to jump out of my skin. Twenty minutes felt like hours. I stuck with it because I was committed to discovering the long-term benefits of the practice, even though, at first, I was very uncomfortable. I didn't have an outcome in mind; I was just curious to experience what, if anything, would change. The changes were subtle, almost imperceptible at first. Over time, I began to feel more and more at ease in the meditation practice, and my sense of time shifted. What at first seemed like hours began to feel like five or ten minutes. But other than the shift in my experience of time, I was unable to explain how the practice was impacting me. Toward the end of the year, I found out. People I didn't know began to give me unsolicited and unexpected feedback about how patient I was. This was startling at first because I had always been so impatient. My son, who is very chill, and I laugh about my attempts to get him to behave like the type A personality I was, even when he was younger. It never worked, but I kept trying anyway. My husband used to tell me to sit down and relax, to no avail. I always claimed that I was too busy. When I began to receive the feedback about how patient I was, I began to notice that I actually had changed. I realized that by intentionally sitting with my impatience for one year, I had actually been transformed. The conditions for this alchemy were consistent practice and surrender. Now, because it is no longer my style, whenever I feel impatient, I know it is a sign that I am stressed and need to slow down, take a breath, and wait until the feeling passes before I say or do anything else.

To learn patience, practice being still. Slow down. Take a moment each day just to notice your breath. Is it fast or slow, deep or shallow? Slow it down. Deepen it. Savor it. Take the time to glimpse a rainbow, smell a rose, hear a baby laugh. When you think you don't have time, tell yourself, "I have all the time in the world." Notice the shift in your perception of time. Achieving a balanced mental outlook and inner peace requires patience. Practicing stillness teaches us that we really do have all the time in the world.

PATIENCE RENEWS

An important practice to develop is the practice of self-renewal. People who are subjected to the ongoing, cumulative, and recurring emotional assaults of ethnic and race-based stress and trauma need to take time out to renew their body, energy, mind, emotions, and psyche. Without renewal, ongoing stress and trauma are overwhelming, taking a toll that leaves you feeling disheartened, drained of energy, and depleted. The Covid-19 global pandemic, coupled with the pandemic of racial violence and injustice, have had a negative impact socially, psychologically, and economically. We can no longer rely on our resilience alone to bounce back from adversity. We need something more. Resilience is the ability to spring back and keep going after hardship, and while it is essential to our health and wellbeing, springing back is not what we are being called to do right now. Collectively, we are in the midst of transformational change, a time when something new wants to be born, a revolution of the heart. I believe we are being called to birth a new consciousness of unconditional love, compassion, wisdom, mercy, and justice for all who are and all that is. This embryo in the womb of consciousness needs to be nurtured, loved, and held so it can grow and develop into its fullness. We don't want to give birth prematurely. We want to give this new consciousness every opportunity to develop fully so that when it is born, it is strong and healthy. Right now, we are being called on to be still, to self-reflect, and to renew. Now is a time to transform the harmful effects of ethnic and race-based traumatic stress that we have endured, and that we have inflicted on others, by cultivating a consciousness that recognizes our innate value, regardless of our skin color, facial features, hair texture, and unique cultural, racial and ethnic identity.

Self-renewal is rebirth and, like any birthing process, is a process that takes time. It requires patience. We are in a season of renewal. During this period of gestation, while we are waiting to give birth to a new consciousness, a means to release old ways of thinking and being, ways that consume our time and deplete our energy, is called for. Now is a time to let go of the stories we tell ourselves that hold us back, like "I'm not enough" or "I'm running out of time" or "I've done something wrong" or "I'm not important" or "I have to say yes because someone asked me to do something." Now is a time to be clear about who you are, and what you value most in life, in yourself and in others. Now is a time to envision the life you want to live and the consciousness you want to occupy. It requires patience to dig deep into your soul to uncover what wants to be birthed in you. Now is the time to rest, reflect, and renew.

REST

Asana/posture

A supported side twist (Salamba Bharadvajasana) is very comforting and supports a sense of ease and timelessness. People who experience ongoing, cumulative, and recurrent race-based stress and trauma need to embody a sense of timelessness and renewal. The inability to rest and renew comes from having an internalized sense that to be still is to be lazy and to prioritize self-care is to be selfish. Practicing a posture like a supported side twist simulates resting in the comfort of a mother's womb where feelings of timelessness and being held in love and cared for are nurtured. Renewal requires patience. For people who have not had the experience of feeling unbound by the restrictions and limitations of linear time, this can be an experience of restoration and revitalization. Affirmations that accompany this pose include "I feel timeless" and "I feel renewed."

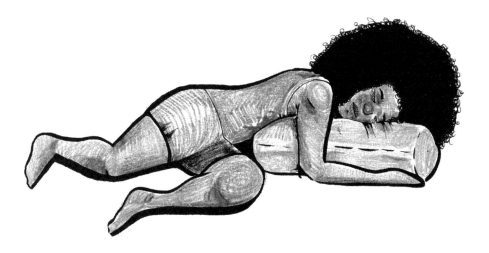

Place your bolster or three rectangular folded blankets stacked on top of each other vertically in the middle of your yoga mat. Sit with your right hip snug up against the narrow end of the bolster. Bend both knees, taking your shins to the left and resting your left ankle in the arch of your right foot. Lift up from your sternum and twist your belly toward the right to square your torso to the front of your mat. Fold over the bolster from this position. Rest your right cheek on the bolster so that your head is facing the same direction as your knees. Keep the back of your neck long and the front of your neck soft. Rest your forearms and hands along the sides of the bolster. Now notice how your breath slows down and deepens. Observe how your inhalations and exhalations root your pelvis and enhance the turning sensation in your belly and shoulders. Do you root more deeply into your pelvis when you inhale or when you exhale? Do you lengthen and move deeper into the twist when you inhale or when you exhale? When you are ready, change sides. Hold this pose for up to 15 minutes on each side. When you are ready to come out of this pose, press both hands into the floor, tuck your chin into your chest, and come up to sitting, lifting your head last.

REFLECT

Affirmations

While in the posture, silently repeat to yourself three times, "Breathing in, I feel timeless... Breathing out, I feel renewed." On your fourth inhale, silently repeat, "Timeless." On your exhale, silently repeat, "Renewed." Continue that repetition—inhale "Timeless," exhale "Renewed"—for at least five more rounds. Rest in this posture, focusing on your breath for up to 15 minutes and then for as long as you are comfortable. When you are ready, change sides and repeat the affirmations on the other side. When you are ready to come out of the pose, take two or three deep diaphragmatic breaths, tuck your chin into your chest, and gently press your hands into the floor to lift back up to sitting.

Repeating the phrases "I feel timeless" and "I feel renewed" plants seeds that can take root in your consciousness and enable you to slow down, take your time, and discover that haste really does make waste. That being patient is powerful. It is a reminder that you really do have all the time in the world. You really do have time to make your health and wellbeing a priority.

RENEW

Journal

In your journal, finish the sentence "I feel timeless and renewed when..."

_____

_____

_____

_____

_____

_____

_____

_____

_____

_____

_____

_____

_____

_____

_____

_____

_____

_____

_____

_____

Journal how this practice benefits you.

_____

_____

_____

_____

_____

_____

_____

_____

_____

_____

_____

_____

_____

_____

_____

_____

_____

_____

_____

_____

_____

Chapter 10

BIRTHING NEW CONSCIOUSNESS

A FARMER and his son had a beloved horse that was considered to be the best horse in town. After years of being groomed and trained by the boy, the horse was more beautiful, more graceful, and ran faster than any other horse in the region. One day upon awakening, the boy and his father discovered that the horse had run away. The boy was heartbroken. When the neighbors gathered to offer their condolences to the farmer for his misfortune, the farmer simply said, "We'll see. We don't know if this is good or if this is bad." A week later, the horse returned with a companion—an equally beautiful wild mare. The boy tamed the mare and the neighbors gathered to celebrate the good fortune of the farmer and his son who now had the two best horses in town. The farmer thanked the villagers and then said, "We don't know if this is good luck or bad luck." Later that day, when the farmer's son was racing the new horse through the fields, he fell off and broke both legs. The village doctor tended to the boy's wounds and then confined him to bed until his legs could heal. The villagers returned to commiserate with the farmer about this unfortunate turn of events. But the farmer, true to form, simply replied by saying, "I am happy that my son is alive. In time his legs will heal. Who knows if his injuries will turn out to be something good or bad?" Within the week, a battalion of soldiers arrived in the village to conscript all of the boys of fighting age to go to war against a neighboring village. The only one left behind was the farmer's son, confined to his bed, because his wounds would take months to heal. The story ends with the farmer looking out across his fields, enjoying the way the sun reflected off the mountain peaks in the distance, gazing at his two fine horses grazing, and feeling happy that his son was safely at home and would not have to go to war.[1]

This Buddhist tale teaches us that good and bad are part of life. They are intertwined. When life gives us what we want, we call it good and we rejoice. When it gives us what we don't want, we call it bad and we complain and lament, just like the villagers in the story. Because of this tendency, we find ourselves on a roller coaster of emotional ups and downs based on how we judge a situation. We cannot always control life's circumstances, but we can control our attitude and our emotional responses to events as they unfold. The farmer's equanimity kept him from becoming caught up in the disappointments, hurts, traumas, and dramas he faced. He understood that nothing lasts forever and he remained open to the possibility contained within each event. In his wisdom, he realized that nothing is ever all good or all bad. He didn't pre-judge the events that took place, nor did he personalize them. He remained open to all of life—the pleasures, the good fortune, the disappointments, and misfortunes that life presented. This openness to all of life's possibilities, both good and bad, helps us remain open to growth opportunities, regardless of what occurs.

Growth is the willingness to be transformed by the process of life as it unfolds before you. Every situation that presents itself is an opportunity for growth. The willingness to find something beneficial in what is typically regarded as being bad keeps you from being stuck in pain and suffering. But here's the catch: your ability to do this doesn't happen automatically. It requires you to sit in your feelings while you go beneath the surface and dig deep enough to discover the growth potential in whatever life brings to bear. It requires the stamina and discipline to tolerate what my father used to refer to as growing pains. Growth is not always easy or pain-free. But the pain of growth is temporary, whereas the refusal or inability to admit to and deal directly with emotionally painful experiences keeps pain locked inside, where it can fester, grow worse, and become chronic. Holding on to pain and suffering stunts your growth. As difficult as it may be to comprehend, much less accept, it is important to recognize that even the worst experiences can help us grow. Three examples of what might typically be regarded as bad experiences that offer growth opportunities are loss, humiliation, and disillusionment. Can you find the growth opportunity inside?

LOSS

Loss is the experience of disconnection. Whether it is the loss of a loved one, a job, your home, a treasured object, your health, respect in your community, or a cherished idea about yourself or someone close to you, no matter how large or how small, temporary or permanent, the experience of loss is painful. We are hardwired for connection, and disconnection born of loss is one of the most emotionally painful experiences a human being suffers. But here's the thing. Loss is a part of life. You cannot change that. What you can change is your attitude about loss. Like the farmer in the story, start considering that loss is not something that happens *to* you; it is just something that happens. Loss is not personal. Your attitude about loss is what's truly important. Loss can help you recognize the value of what has been lost as well as the value of what you are left with. It is sometimes through the loss of a relationship, possession, your health, or other circumstance that you learn to appreciate those things you normally take for granted. Something as simple, for example, as your breath. You don't usually think about the value of being able to breathe effortlessly until your breathing is compromised. There is a story in the Chandogya Upanishad 5.1.6–15 that illustrates what loss can teach us.

> A competition breaks out between the five yogic senses: mind, breath, speech, hearing, and sight. Each sense maintains that it is the most important of all the senses, and wants to be recognized as such. To discover which of the senses is most important, they decide that each one will leave the body in turn to see who is most missed. Speech leaves first, and although mute, the body lives on. Sight leaves next, and although blind, the body survives. Then hearing leaves, and although deaf, the body perseveres. Next the mind leaves, and although it is no longer very smart, life persists. Finally, breath leaves the body. Naturally, the body immediately begins to die. "Wait! Stop! Come back! Come back!" clamor the other senses. Breath returns to be heralded ever after as supreme among the yogic senses.[2]

The temporary loss of breath heightened the awareness of its importance.

In the instance of what appears to be a permanent loss, you can still recover and grow. I emphasize "what appears" to be a permanent loss because when you open to it, embrace it, and accept it instead of resisting it, loss can take you deeper into your heart and reveal something invaluable. I was 30 years old when my mother died. I mourned her loss and missed her terribly for many years. But over time, missing her transformed into beautiful, wonderful memories of her that continue to fill my heart with great joy. At times, I still wish that she was with me physically, but blessedly I have discovered that she is always with me in my heart. As the years go by, I love her more than ever, and for this I am grateful. Losing my mother taught me that love lives on in the heart even when the person is no longer physically present. Loss taught me that the energy of love itself is what is constant, not the physical existence of a loved one.

Loss can also open you to the blessing of possibility, as it did for three war veterans: one veteran of the Vietnam war, one veteran of the Iraq war, and one veteran of the Afghanistan war. Two of the veterans lost both their legs in combat, and one lost one of his legs. In spite of their significant loss, in April 2010 the three of them together, with only one leg between them, successfully climbed 19,340 feet to the highest peak of Mount Kilimanjaro in Tanzania. To paraphrase them, *no matter what loss you have experienced you can still accept challenge, which opens you to the blessing of possibility.*[3]

HUMILIATION

Humiliation is an intentional and essential ingredient in the recipe of racial wounding. It is the attempt to exercise power over others to make them feel inferior. It is always abusive. It can take many different forms—ridicule, scolding, derision, and physical abuse are a few examples. Whether you are the one being humiliated or the one observing humiliation, it is painful. When I was a little girl, I remember feeling humiliated whenever I saw images of Black actors in movies and on television being depicted as buffoons, victims, villains, or as being subservient. This was especially painful because at the time these were the only images of Black actors being portrayed. As a child, I knew nothing about stereotypes and racist tropes. What I did know was that the images on the screen were degrading and that I felt repulsed and ashamed when I saw them. I was confused because I didn't know if the shame I felt was of myself, of the images, or of the feelings of repulsion I experienced watching people who I identified with being degraded. As a child, I internalized and personalized the images I saw and that was painful. I didn't know at the time that those negative portrayals were shameful depictions that intentionally portrayed

Black and other non-White people as inferior: think Charlie Chan, a Chinese detective played by a Swedish actor made up to "look" Chinese; Tonto (a name that means stupid), the Native American sidekick of the Lone Ranger, a White American, heroic cowboy; and Stepin Fetchit, Hollywood's first Black actor who famously intoned, "Feets don't fail me now," and played a mumbling, confused, subservient buffoon afraid of everything, especially ghosts. I know now that the shame I felt as a child actually belongs to the perpetrators of those negative depictions, not to the ones being depicted or the ones watching the depictions. But those images left lifelong impressions that can still trigger memories of the deep emotional wounding they inflicted. I cannot help but wonder what impressions they left on the White children viewing those images.

When it comes to feeling humiliated, one size does not fit all. Everyone does not feel humiliated by the same things. What humiliates you may be totally insignificant to someone else. But the feeling of shame that is triggered by humiliating experiences is universal. Make no mistake: when you are being humiliated, it is not because of anything you have done wrong; it is because you are being wronged. The pain you feel is a normal response to being hurt. Even though humiliation is painful, it invites you into a deeper contemplation of your true value. When you go within and reflect on the humiliating experience, you will likely discover that the feelings of shame and embarrassment you feel are not because you are inferior or deserving of the humiliation, but because of someone else's need to exercise power over you in order to feel superior. Knowing that is empowering.

Humiliating experiences can teach you that what other people think of you is none of your business. Your business is to determine what you think of yourself. What do you value about you? The more you focus on valuing yourself, the less vulnerable you are to feeling humiliated. What you focus on expands. If you have a hard time identifying what you value about yourself, start by repeating this affirmation: "I love and approve of myself." "I love and approve of myself." "I love and approve of myself."

DISILLUSIONMENT
Disillusionment is difficult because it challenges your belief system, your values, and your assumptions. It is the recognition that everything is not what it appears to be or what you thought it was. At first, this can be disorienting

and can result in a temporary state of anxiety and or depression. But if you make the effort to go deeper, you can get beyond the anxiety and depression you feel and can realize the benefits of disillusionment. In the musical *The Wiz*, an adaptation of *The Wizard of Oz*, the characters in the story embark on a perilous journey in search of the Wiz, an unknown, unseen mythological source, who they hoped would grant them their deepest heart's desires. After encountering much danger and overcoming obstacles along the way, they finally reached their destination. When they met with the Wiz face to face, they were astonished, angry, and disappointed to discover that his so-called power was a figment of their imaginations. It was only then that they realized the power they had attributed to him was actually power they already possessed. They had within themselves what they had been seeking all along. Disillusionment allowed the Tin Man to see that he already had a heart; the Scarecrow to realize that he already had a brain; the Cowardly Lion to recognize that he already had courage; and Dorothy realized that no external search can help you find your heart's desire. Disillusionment can help you see that you already are who you're trying to become and that everything you need lies within you—you just need to believe it to see it. Disillusionment can help you believe in your own gifts and power.

THANK YOU, I THINK

Remember, every situation is an opportunity for growth. So when you encounter loss, humiliation, or disillusionment, look for the growth opportunity hidden in these hurtful experiences. Consider that these experiences may actually be blessings in disguise. When you are in the midst of any of these experiences, it's hard to perceive anything good about them. And make no mistake, it is not the loss, the humiliating event, or the disillusionment that is good; it is the growth potential inside loss, humiliation, and disillusionment that is good. Just try to remember that loss can help you realize that the person who leaves you lives on in your heart. The cherished object you lose can teach you the valuable lesson of letting go or of non-attachment, and making room for something new. The loss of a physical ability, financial stability, or even your home can teach you that the world has not come to an end and that you have the inner resources and resilience to bounce back to meet the challenges you face. Humiliation can teach you to stop caring about what others think of you and to care more about what you think of yourself. As painful as humiliation can be, it can empower you to shift from an external to an internal focus and to stop shaming, blaming, or criticizing yourself for someone else's abusive behavior. Disillusionment helps you see with more clarity. You are better able to see reality as it is, not as you imagined it to be. In *The Wiz*, disillusionment taught the Tin Man, the Cowardly Lion, the Scarecrow, and Dorothy to believe in themselves—they already had everything they needed if they just looked within.

The Universe in its infinite wisdom has a way of providing you with opportunities for growth through life lessons. Every day it provides you with opportunities to become more loving, patient, and kind, and to rid yourself of anger, jealousy, and fear. Sometimes, because you may be slow to get the message, the lesson may show up over and over again until you get the point. It may take years for you to figure out what the lesson is in the hardship you experience, much less what it has to offer. But even if the lesson eludes you, you still want to look for it. You may not choose the hardships you face, but the way you engage hardship or challenge is always a matter of choice. If you're not quite ready to say thank you for the hidden blessings to be found in loss, humiliation, or disillusionment, maybe you can start with thank you, I think.

POST-TRAUMATIC GROWTH

Post-traumatic growth is defined as a person's ability to regroup after experiencing a traumatic event, and to experience shifts in consciousness that result in positive, transformational change. It involves the ability to find the growth opportunity hidden in the stressful series of traumatic events that one experiences. Post-traumatic growth occurs when you are able to find meaning in your pain and suffering, and to emerge with a greater sense of purpose. It is different from resilience, which is the ability to bounce back from stress and trauma. Post-traumatic growth refers to the ability to reconstruct or rebuild a meaningful, purposeful life after everything one previously believed falls apart. Occasionally, growth after trauma happens in a spontaneous, sudden moment of insight, an aha moment, but that is not usually the case. Typically, it doesn't happen without effort that involves deep inner reflection and soul searching. But at some point after experiencing trauma, it is possible to experience personal growth, enjoy better relationships, gain a greater appreciation for life in general, and to have a spiritual awakening. Traumatic events change us. After trauma, we are no longer the person we were. I remember a client who was the lone survivor of a fatal car crash, who was severely injured, and whose doctors were surprised that she survived. When she came for therapy, she said, "I've become a new girl and I want you to help me get to know her." That awareness and her acceptance of the way she had been changed by her experience are examples of post-traumatic growth trying to happen. But it did not happen overnight, and she had to be willing to heal from her trauma and make the necessary effort in order to grow.

In her book *The Salt Eaters*, Toni Cade Bambara tells the story of Velma, a burnt-out community activist who attempted suicide after becoming exhausted, depressed, and disillusioned with her fight for civil rights and equal justice, and her constant battle against oppression. Her failed suicide attempt leads her to seek healing at the community health center that she helped to establish. Minnie, an aged faith healer, is called in to work on Velma. The story begins with Minnie asking Velma, "Are you sure, sweetheart, that you want to be well? … Just so's you're sure, sweetheart, and ready to be healed, cause wholeness is no trifling matter. A lot of weight when you're well."[4] To grow, we cannot remain stuck in the prison of our pain.

Growth can be facilitated by reimagining yourself, your future, and the world. There are numerous examples of those who have turned a tragic life event or a lifetime of stress and trauma into a life of meaning and purpose. Parents who have lost loved ones to gun violence are examples. After her 17-year-old son was shot and killed by a man who was enraged that her son and his friends were playing music too loudly in their car, Lucy McBath left her job as a flight attendant and ran for public office and was elected to the United States Congress. She joined other African American mothers whose sons were murdered to form an organization called Mothers of the Movement. She became an advocate for gun control and has dedicated her life to preventing others, regardless of race or ethnicity, from having the same experience she had. She used the tragedy to create meaning and purpose in the face of one of the most traumatic events a person can experience: the death of a child. She made her experience bigger than herself and her personal loss.

Another example of post-traumatic growth is the story of two young men who were arrested in a neighborhood coffee shop when they declined to place an order while they waited for a business associate to arrive for a pre-arranged meeting. The store manager called the police who handcuffed and arrested the young men. They were detained for nine hours. No criminal charges were filed because they had not committed a crime. As devastating and humiliating as the experience was, in a televised interview the two young men said they would use this event as an opportunity to make something positive come out of it, and to inspire others who might be subjected to the kind of harassment they experienced. They did just that. The men agreed to work with the city and a nonprofit organization where the incident occurred to develop criteria, review applications, and establish a pilot curriculum for public high school students to develop the skills necessary to pursue their dream of being entrepreneurs.[5] We don't always hear the stories, but there is a long history of these kinds of examples of determination to use encounters of racial harassment, violence, and trauma for personal and community growth.

HEALING NARRATIVES

Part of our growth involves learning to tell healing stories of love for ourselves, our families, and our communities, so that eventually these positive and uplifting stories become the norm and the lens through which we view ourselves. It's easy to get stuck telling stories of hardship, pain, and suffering because it is real and prevalent. But it's important to remember that we are so much more than our stories of pain and suffering. While those stories are very real, they are only a part of us, and we do not have to be defined by them. When we become overly identified with our pain, we lose touch with our triumphs, our joys, our creativity, and our strengths. Remember, what we focus on expands.

To facilitate post-traumatic growth in ourselves, we need to create and then share with each other new and healing narratives—stories of our own heroism, perseverance, and triumph in overcoming the obstacles that living in a racialized culture imposes. This is different from reading *about* the heroism, strength, creativity, and the genius of our heroes and sheroes. This is about crafting and sharing narratives of our own courage. People exposed to ongoing, recurrent, and cumulative race-based stress and trauma have always done what is necessary to move beyond surviving. We have worked hard to improve and change our circumstances so we could thrive. We have done so by working in collaboration with others, but we have had to call on our perseverance, resourcefulness, and resilience to thrive. Even when the obstacles that block the way to equal opportunity and equal treatment under the law seem impossible to surmount, we have taken inspiration and strength from our families, from our communities, from a higher power, from the past, from the stories of other people, and from within ourselves to make a way out of no way. Each one of us can be a model for others who feel oppressed and defeated by obstacles that seem insurmountable. I learned from my father who showed my brother and me how to persevere even when it seemed there was no way to overcome the obstacles we faced. I'll share his story with you. His story is a story of triumph. His story is our story. It belongs to all of us.

He never wanted to make history, he just wanted to fly. My father, Frederick L. Parker, Jr., was born June 25, 1920, the third of six children. While he was raised on the Southside of Chicago, his parents owned a farm in Cassopolis, Michigan, where the family spent summer vacations. During his youth, he loved nothing more than spending lazy summer afternoons lying on his back, gazing toward the sky in the meadow near the farmhouse. Hands cupped over his forehead like an awning shielding his eyes from the sun, he watched birds flying overhead, soaring, dipping, and diving for hours at a time. What freedom, he thought. He tried to imagine what it would be like to be as free as those birds. My father's dream was to one day become an aviator.

When he graduated from junior college, because he was not yet 21, he had to get his father's permission to enlist in the Illinois National Guard and attend officer candidate school. He was later commissioned as a Second Lieutenant in the United States Army Air Corps. In 1943, he attended pilot training at Tuskegee Airfield in Alabama as part of an "experiment" to train African American fighter pilots. Graduates of his class of 1944 were an integral part of the infamous 332nd fighter group called the Red-Tail Angels.

At that time, the United States armed forces were racially segregated. The military propaganda was that African American pilots were unfit for anything but the lowest ranks of military service. An infamous report issued by the war college in 1925 stated that Black pilots were not smart enough or disciplined enough to fly combat aircraft. The pilot training program, known as the Tuskegee Experiment, was in actuality designed to prove that the military propaganda of the day was factual.

However, in spite of the obstacles they faced, these men refused to accept the limitations others tried to impose on them. To them, every obstacle they faced was just another door in the way. The Red-Tails flew hundreds of successful missions as bomber escorts over North Africa and Europe, eventually gaining the respect and admiration of the military brass—the same people who questioned their ability and doubted their courage.

Rather than chasing after and downing enemy aircraft for their own personal glory, these pilots had a reputation for staying with the bombers they were assigned to safeguard. They risked their own lives, to protect the lives of others as they flew through enemy territory. Once they appeared as escorts, the bomber pilots and crews knew without a doubt that they would be protected from enemy fighters. It is a matter of record: the Red-Tail Angels lost fewer bombers than any other bomber escorts during the war.

The Tuskegee Airmen fought a war on two fronts. They helped to destroy Adolf Hitler's regime, defeating Nazi tyranny. At the same time they helped end racial segregation in the United States armed services—all because they wanted the freedom to fly, and the freedom to fight for their country. In the process, they helped to end oppression abroad as well as at home. They weren't trying to make history; *they were trying to make a difference.* By remaining true to their heart's deepest desires and to their calling, they changed the world.

As far as I know, my father never once stepped onto a yoga mat. Yet it is through his example that I learned what living yoga off the yoga mat really means. It's about attitudes and actions that keep you focused, calm, and non-reactive in the face of life's challenges. It's about doing what's right, not what's easy. He did this by valiantly fighting for freedoms, at his own peril, that were not always granted to him, because it was the right thing to do. He demonstrated courage by standing up for and insisting on equal treatment for all, even in the face of overwhelming opposition. He proved that obstacles are overcome by committing to relentlessly follow your heart's deepest desires, no matter who or what opposes you. He demonstrated that living life heroically means living life authentically and facing your fears head on, every day, with an open heart.

He lived a life of activism and helped to change the world.

- To live life fully, we are called on to live a life of service to others. Ask yourself each day upon awakening, what difference you want to make in someone else's life. It doesn't have to be a monumental difference. It could be something as simple as offering a listening ear to a friend in need, making a phone call to someone you've been thinking about, or running an errand for a neighbor.

- Rather than focusing on what you may be getting out of a relationship or a situation, shift your focus to what you have to give and offer that. Do this without the expectation of a return.
- Do not let limitations or barriers keep you from pursuing your dreams. No achievement comes without obstacles. Just keep putting one foot in front of the other and continue moving toward your goal. Remember, no effort you make goes unrewarded. Keep looking for a job if you're unemployed. Keep applying to schools until you're admitted. Finish what you start. Don't give up.
- When you know someone has been wronged or treated unfairly, instead of looking the other way, for fear of others' disapproval, stand up for what you know is right.

You may never be called upon to put your life on the line for a person, a cause, or a purpose, but we are all called on to live our lives authentically. Only you and you alone can know what that means, but whatever it means to you, find the courage to be true to it. An authentic life is a life well lived. It is possible to experience growth from adversity and become a better person because of it. My father always said, "Where there's life, there's hope." When the barriers you face seem too difficult to overcome, I hope you will remember his words and his example.

REST

Asana/posture

Supported reclining bound angle pose (Supta Baddha Konasana) is a pose that reminds me of giving birth. Our yoga practice supports birthing new consciousness, so I select it as a final posture, as a means of sealing whatever shifts in consciousness have occurred during the practice. The pose teaches that there is safety and a sense of relief in letting go of trying to control what one cannot control, and to instead allow stillness and silence to do its work; it involves surrender. It gives practitioners an opportunity to experience the body's ability to restore and repair, and to support resilience, health, and growth without any other assistance. It allows us to get out of the way and let the body take good care of us. It supports remembered wellness. The affirmations that accompany this pose are "I feel whole" and "I feel complete."

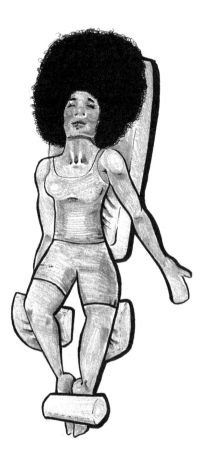

Place a bolster or a narrow stack of three rectangular folded blankets vertically in the middle of your yoga mat. Place an additional folded blanket or a neck pillow at the top of your bolster to support your head or your neck. The lower edge of the blankets or bolster should come directly into contact with your buttocks to support your lower back. Bring the soles of your feet together, touching as if in a prayer position, and, if you like, place a small pillow across your feet, then spread your knees apart. Each knee fanned out to the side is supported by a yoga block, blanket roll, meditation cushion, or bolsters. Lower yourself onto your back over the bolster. If you like, cover your eyes with an eye pillow and cover your body with a blanket. Breathe deeply and surrender to gravity as you relax. This pose should be held for a minimum of five minutes and can be held for up to 20 minutes.

REFLECT

Affirmations

While in the posture, silently repeat to yourself three times, "Breathing in, I feel whole... Breathing out, I feel complete." On your fourth inhale, silently repeat, "Whole." On your exhale, silently repeat, "Complete." Continue that repetition—inhale "Whole," exhale "Complete"—for at least five more rounds. To come out of the pose, lift your knees off the support, bringing both knees back to center, place the soles of your feet on the floor, and roll off the bolster onto your right side, coming into fetal position. Pause here for five to ten breaths and enjoy your breath. To come out of the pose, tuck your chin into your chest and use the strength of your arms to lift into a sitting position.

Repeating the phrases "I feel whole" and "I feel complete" plants seeds that can take root in your consciousness and enable you to experience the fullness of your being. While your pain and suffering are real, and need to be acknowledged and healed, you are so much more than your pain and suffering. You also have gifts and talents, triumphs and accomplishments, joys and aspirations. You are multidimensional. This pose supports you in accepting all of who you are.

RENEW

Journal

In your journal, finish the sentence "I feel whole and complete when..."

_____

_____

_____

_____

_____

_____

_____

_____

_____

_____

_____

_____

_____

_____

_____

_____

_____

_____

_____

_____

_____

Journal how this practice benefits you.

_____

_____

_____

_____

_____

_____

_____

_____

_____

_____

_____

_____

_____

_____

_____

_____

_____

_____

_____

_____

_____

_____

Epilogue

WHEN WE try to change something for the better without self-reflective awareness, or when we are in too great a hurry, we miss recognizing the pitfalls and perils of the actions we are taking and create more pain and suffering.

I've told the story of being the only person of color in a yoga class when the hip hop music the yoga teacher selected for her playlist included the "n" word and no one appeared to notice but me. Rather than reacting in the moment, I remember silently repeating to myself, "Do not have an outburst. Do not have an outburst. Do not have an outburst." I used the rest of the class to decide what I would say to the teacher after class. When I confronted her, the teacher claimed that she didn't hear the lyric, smiled apologetically, and said, "I'm sorry." After class, no one made eye contact with me, and then someone asked me why I had to say something to the teacher in front of the entire class, as if my speaking up was the problem. The studio owner apologized, applauded me for speaking out, removed the teacher from teaching the class, and asked her to call me to extend another apology. Then she asked if there was anything else that needed to be done to make me feel comfortable enough to return to the studio. There was nothing more she could have said or done. The damage was done. I no longer felt safe and did not want to return.

It was inconceivable to me that the teacher didn't hear the lyrics on the playlist she created. I was positive that she heard the lyrics and selected the music anyway, and that the rest of the class intentionally ignored or denied what they heard. "How is it possible that she didn't hear the 'n' word?" I wondered. "I heard it, so she *must* have heard it," I told myself. "The rest of the class must have heard it too. If they didn't hear it, why not? Why am I the only one speaking up?" We are meaning-making beings and the stories we tell ourselves help us make sense of the world and help us derive meaning from the events that take place in our lives. Our stories are subjective and tend to match our life experience and whatever emotional state we're in at the time the narrative emerges. Here's how it works. First your nervous system reacts to a situation. You feel it in your body. When I heard the "n" word, I felt like I'd been punched in the gut. Next, your brain makes up a story to match your nervous system's response. "If I heard the 'n' word, then the teacher did too. She chose to play the music anyway, lied about not hearing the lyric, and the rest of the class chose to ignore what they heard." Then the story triggers an emotional reaction. I felt angry and betrayed. Finally, you take action. I decided to speak up and to stop attending classes at the studio. The sequence of cascading reactions I describe happened automatically. The only conscious choices I made were to speak up and to stop taking classes at the studio.

We filter information and interpret events through our own lived experience. That's why every event that occurs does not have the same impact on you and why there can be several different interpretations of the same event. Your interpretation of an event is not the same as the event itself, but when you're not aware of that it's easy to conflate your interpretations with the facts of the event, and to assume that you are seeing things clearly. We rarely have an immediate or direct sense that our perceptions are clouded or wrong, and when you habitually regard your interpretations as factual, without self-reflective awareness, you can make errors in judgment that can lead to serious and sometimes deadly consequences. Think about police officers who murder unarmed Black people and claim it's because they fear for their lives. Are they reacting to an external threat or an internal trigger? What is the story they're telling themselves? Did you hear about the woman who called the police to report that she was endangered by a Black man, when all he did was ask her to follow a city ordinance by asking her to put a leash on her dog in a public park? And recall the example from Chapter 10 of the store manager who called the police when two Black men declined to place an order while they waited for someone to join them in a coffee shop? What was the story they were telling themselves? Were their interpretations of danger accurate or clouded by an accumulation of habitual, unconscious ways of perceiving and behaving?[1]

Interpretation is not the same as observation. Interpretation is your guess about what you observe. Yoga teaches us that our interpretation of an event can be clouded by certain obstacles that prevent us from seeing clearly. The Yoga Sutra uses the term avidya[2] to describe the four obstacles that lead to misperceptions or misapprehension; our ego needs (asmita), our attachments (raga), our aversions (dvesa), and our fears (abhinivesa). Misapprehension is regarded as the root of behaviors that lead to more pain and suffering. Yoga practices invite us to occupy the seat of awareness, to slow our minds down, reflect on our thoughts and feelings, and gain clarity so that we can exercise discernment before we take action. Regardless of race or ethnicity, awareness is the first step toward healing race-based traumatic stress. When you're operating with awareness, you're able to tell the difference between your observation of an event and your interpretation of the event. The story I was telling myself was my interpretation, not my observation. Confusing the story I was telling myself with the observation was problematic. In actuality, I had no idea why the teacher did what she did or why the rest of the class remained silent, but I was convinced that I knew. As long as I clung to the story I was telling myself (raga) about what happened as factual—"the teacher was lying and the students didn't care about what they heard"—I was unable to process the event with awareness. Even though I exercised restraint and was measured in my response, as long as I remained stuck in my story, I was trapped in feeling angry and hurt. Holding on to the story without further examining it interfered with my ability to process the event in a way that could lead to growth. Luckily for me, I don't like feeling stuck in hurt and anger, so I kept up my efforts to heal from the experience by continuing to reflect on it, even though that was sometimes painful. The growing pains of discomfort should not be confused with the pain caused by misapprehension. When we engage in self-reflective awareness, we become sensitive to our own suffering and its causes, as well as to the pain and suffering we cause others. It is the awareness of our pain and suffering that alerts us to the fact that something is wrong. Awareness is the first step toward freeing ourselves.

Each moment and every event holds within it an infinite number of possible reactions and responses. With awareness, you begin to realize that, and rather than clinging to and acting on your interpretations, or remaining stuck in your pain and suffering, you consider other possibilities. This is not to say that you bypass, overlook, or make excuses for what has occurred. You don't. In my case, what happened actually did occur. The teacher's playlist did include the "n" word. The teacher did deny that she heard the lyric. The people in the class did remain silent. I did feel hurt, angry, and betrayed. That's the observation. The interpretation was the story I told myself about what occurred. I credit my yoga practice with my ability to resist having an outburst when I heard the offensive "n" word lyric, and to instead pause, reflect, and think about how I wanted to respond. I credit my practice with my ability to eventually separate out the incident from the story I told myself about the incident, and my willingness to be curious about and reflect on why I continued to be so angry and hurt about what happened long after the event. My commitment to self-study, svadhyaya,[3] an important aspect of any yoga practice, eventually led to a surprising insight I had never considered before. What if the teacher was telling the truth? What if she hadn't heard the lyric? What if I actually was the only one who heard it? What if the teacher and students didn't register the lyric because of their oblivion and/or indifference to issues of race? What if they didn't speak up because of what we now call "white fragility," a symptom of their own unacknowledged and unhealed racial wounds? None of these possibilities changed what had occurred, but they offered a perspective that expanded my consciousness and challenged my initial assumptions. It was a transformational moment for me that actually led me to the work I am doing today: bringing awareness to the fact that racial stress and trauma affect all people, not just Black, Brown and Indigenous people; that "white fragility" is a symptom of unhealed racial wounds; and that yoga has the potential to transform the emotional injury of ongoing, recurrent, and cumulative race-based traumatic stress.

We each have our own unique response to the stresses and traumas associated with racial insensitivity, discrimination, injustice, and violence, and our own unique way of recovering. When we are able to process our trauma with awareness, we can grow from the experience. You cannot rush the process of growth, but you can engage in self-study and self-care practices that support growth—practices that involve rest, reflection, and renewal. But it's important to understand that transforming the ongoing, recurrent, cumulative impact of race-based traumatic stress is not something you do overnight, or once and for all. It takes time and requires an ongoing process involving self-reflective awareness, a willingness to transform, as well as daily practices that help you remain resilient and strong.

My hope is that the practices in this guidebook will support you in letting go of your attachment to the stories of pain and suffering you are telling yourself, the ones you identify with, not because your stories aren't real—they are—but because you are so much more than your stories of pain and suffering. We know that suffering exists, but clinging to rather than processing our stories keeps us stuck and prevents post-traumatic growth. This guide is intended to offer a pathway to processing and transforming race-based traumatic stress into growth opportunities that you can model and then share with others. This is how we change the world. The stories we tell ourselves matter. Do the stories you tell yourself help you grow? You always have the power to create new and healing narratives. What are the new and healing stories you choose to tell?

REFERENCES

PROLOGUE

1   Parker, G. (2020) *Restorative Yoga for Ethnic and Race-Based Stress and Trauma*. London/ Philadelphia: Singing Dragon.

INTRODUCTION

1   Aziz, S. (2020, April 12) "Anti-Asian racism must be stopped before it is normalised." *Al Jazeera*. Accessed on 02/25/2021 at www.aljazeera.com/indepth/opinion/anti-asian-racism-stopped-normalised-200412103717485.html

2   Al Jazeera (2020, April 12) "African nationals 'mistreated, evicted' in China over coronavirus." *Al Jazeera*. Accessed on 02/25/2021 at www.aljazeera.com/news/2020/04/african-students-mistreated-evicted-china-coronavrus-200412100315200.html

3   Pinsker, J. (2020, April 10) "The pandemic will cleave America in two." *The Atlantic*. Accessed on 02/25/2021 at www.theatlantic.com/family/archive/2020/04/two-pandemics-us-coronavirus-inequality/609622

4   Eligon, J. (2020, April 7) "Black Americans face alarming rates of coronavirus infection in some states." *The New York Times*. Accessed on 02/25/2021 at www.nytimes.com/2020/04/07/us/coronavirus-race.html

5   Smedley, B.S. (2003) *Unequal Treatment: Confronting Racial and Ethnic Disparities in Health Care*. Washington, DC: National Academies Press.

6   Harknes, J. (Director) (2008) *Game of Change* [Motion picture]. USA.

7   Jernigan, M.M., Green, C.E., Pérez-Gualdrón, L., Liu, M. *et al.* (2015) "#racialtraumaisreal." Institute for the Study and Promotion of Race and Culture. Accessed on 02/25/2021 at www.bc.edu/content/dam/bc1/schools/lsoe/sites/isprc/racialtraumaisreal.pdf

8   Jernigan, M.M., Green, C.E., Pérez-Gualdrón, L., Liu, M. *et al.* (2015) "#racialtraumaisreal." Institute for the Study and Promotion of Race and Culture. Accessed on 02/25/2021 at www.bc.edu/content/dam/bc1/schools/lsoe/sites/isprc/racialtraumaisreal.pdf

9   Stahl, J.E., Dossett, M.L., LaJoie, A.S., Denninger, J.W. *et al.* (2015, October 13) "Relaxation response and resiliency training and its effects on healthcare resource utilization." *PLoS ONE 10*, 10. doi:10.1371/journal.pone.0140212

10 Moore, C. (2019, April 7) "Positive daily affirmations: Is there science behind it?" Positive-Psychology. Accessed on 02/25/2021 at https://positivepsychology.com/daily-affirmations

11 Pennebaker, J. (2004) *Writing to Heal: A Guided Journal for Recovering from Trauma and Emotional Upheaval.* Oakland, CA: New Harbinger Publications.

12 Woods-Giscombé, C.L. and Gaylord, S.A. (2014, January 17) "The cultural relevance of mindfulness meditation as a health intervention for African Americans: Implications for reducing stress-related health disparities." *Journal of Holistic Nursing 32*, 3.

13 Benson, H. (2000) *The Relaxation Response.* New York, NY: HarperCollins.

14 Desikachar, T. (1999) *The Heart of Yoga: Developing a Personal Practice.* Rochester, VT: Inner Traditions International.

CHAPTER 2

1   Harris, A. (2017, April 6) "Against spanking: Stacey Patton, author of new book about black America's relationship with corporal punishment, says it's time to understand it as abuse, not mere discipline." *Slate.* Accessed on 02/25/2021 at https://slate.com/human-interest/2017/04/its-time-for-black-america-to-stop-spanking-its-kids-says-author-stacey-patton.html

2   Green, A. (2017, June 29) "How black girls aren't presumed to be innocent." *The Atlantic.* Accessed on 02/25/2021 at www.theatlantic.com/politics/archive/2017/06/black-girls-innocence-georgetown/532050

3   Goff, P.A. (2014, February 24) "Black boys viewed as older, less innocent than whites, research finds." American Psychological Association. Accessed on 02/25/2021 at www.apa.org/news/press/releases/2014/03/black-boys-older

4   Flores, A. (2015, January 6) "Everything we know about the Tamar Rice shooting investigation." *BuzzFeedNews.* Accessed on 02/25/2021 at www.buzzfeednews.com/article/alisonvingiano/everything-we-know-tamir-rice

5   Maxouris, C.M. (2020, August 27) "Kenosha shooting suspect faces more homicide charges." *CNN.* Accessed on 02/25/2021 at www.cnn.com/2020/08/27/us/kenosha-wisconsin-shooting-suspect/index.html

6   Bradsher, K. (1999, November 17) "Michigan boy who killed at 11 is convicted of murder as adult." *The New York Times.* Accessed on 02/25/2021 at www.nytimes.com/1999/11/17/us/michigan-boy-who-killed-at-11-is-convicted-of-murder-as-adult.html

7   Cohen, J.S. (2020, July 14) "A teenager didn't do her online schoolwork. So a judge sent her to juvenile detention." ProPublica Illinois. Accessed on 02/25/2021 at www.propublica. org/article/a-teenager-didnt-do-her-online-schoolwork-so-a-judge-sent-her-to-juvenile-detention

8   Khandare, V.A. (2013, August) "Mapping color and caste discrimination in Indian society." Accessed on 02/25/2021 at www.researchgate.net/publication/285414433_Mapping_Color_and_Caste_Discrimination_in_Indian_Society

9   Sunder, L. (2015, November 7) "The Indian caste system and karma theory." *The Shade.* Accessed on 02/25/2021 at https://medium.com/@literose/the-indian-caste-system-and-karma-theory-3327d35664f

CHAPTER 3

1   Kornfield, J. (2002) *The Art of Forgiveness, Loving Kindness, and Peace.* New York, NY: Bantam Dell, p.25.

CHAPTER 4

1   Clifton, L. (1974) "the thirty eighth year." *The Collected Poems of Lucille Clifton.* Copyright © 1974, 1987 by Lucille Clifton. Reprinted with the permission of The Permissions Company, LLC on behalf of BOA Editions, Ltd., boaeditions.org.

2   Lewis, J. (2020, July 30) "Together, you can redeem the soul of our nation." *The New York Times.* Accessed on 02/25/2021 at www.nytimes.com/2020/07/30/opinion/john-lewis-civil-rights-america.html

CHAPTER 5

1   Williams, C. (2020, June 26) "You want a Confederate monument? My body is a Confederate monument." *The New York Times.* Accessed on 02/25/2021 at www.nytimes.com/2020/06/26/opinion/confederate-monuments-racism.html

CHAPTER 6

1   Northrup, S. (2014) *Twelve Years a Slave* (ed. D. Wilson). Vancouver, BC: Engage Books.

2   Desikachar, T.K.V. (1999) *The Heart of Yoga: Developing a Personal Practice.* Rochester, VT: Inner Traditions International, p.171. Sutra 2.18 and 2.20.

CHAPTER 8

1 Bracey, H.R., Rosenblum, J., Sanford, A., and Trueblood, R. (1990) *Managing from the Heart*. New York, NY: Dell Publishing.

2 HEART acronym adapted from Bracey, H., Rosenblum, J., Sanford, A., and Trueblood, R. (1990) *Managing from the Heart*. New York, NY: Dell Publishing, p.189.

CHAPTER 9

1 Augustine of Hippo, St. (n.d.) "Augustine of Hippo." Goodreads. Accessed on 02/25/2021 at www.goodreads.com/author/show/6819578.Augustine_of_Hippo

CHAPTER 10

1 Adapted from the Buddhist tale "The Horse That Got Away" in Conover, S. (2010) *Kindness: A Treasury of Buddhist Wisdom for Children and Parents*. Boston, MA: Skinner House Books.

2 Parker, G. (2020) *Restorative Yoga for Ethnic and Race-Based Stress and Trauma*. London/Philadelphia: Singing Dragon.

3 Associated Press (2010, August 12). "3 war veteran amputees climb Kilimanjaro with one good leg among them." *Deseret News*. Accessed on 02/25/2021 at www.deseret.com/2010/8/12/20133862/3-war-veteran-amputees-climb-kilimanjaro-with-one-good-leg-among-them

4 Bambara, T.C. (1980) *The Salt Eaters*. New York, NY: Random House.

5 Pomrenze, P.S. and Simon, D. (2018, May 2) "Black men arrested at Philadelphia Starbucks reach agreements." *CNN*. Accessed on 02/25/2021 at www.cnn.com/2018/05/02/us/starbucks-arrest-agreements/index.html

EPILOGUE

1 In yoga, habitually unconscious, repetitive behavior is called samskara. For more information, refer to Parker, G. (2020) *Restorative Yoga for Ethnic and Race-Based Stress and Trauma*. London/Philadelphia: Singing Dragon, pp.105–108.

2 For a more detailed discussion of avidya, refer to Parker, G. (2020) *Restorative Yoga for Ethnic and Race-Based Stress and Trauma*. London/Philadelphia: Singing Dragon, pp.137–139.

3 For more detail on svadhyaya, refer to Parker, G. (2020) *Restorative Yoga for Ethnic and Race-Based Stress and Trauma*. London/Philadelphia: Singing Dragon, pp.211–213.